Basics of Mechanical Ventilation

Hooman Poor

Basics of Mechanical Ventilation

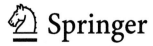 Springer

Hooman Poor
Mount Sinai – National Jewish Health Respiratory Institute
Icahn School of Medicine
New York, NY
USA

ISBN 978-3-319-89980-0   ISBN 978-3-319-89981-7   (eBook)
https://doi.org/10.1007/978-3-319-89981-7

Library of Congress Control Number: 2018944605

Printed on acid-free paper

This Springer imprint is published by the registered company Springer
International Publishing AG part of Springer Nature
The registered company address is: Gewerbestrasse 11, 6330 Cham, Switzerland

Dedicated to Conner, Ellery, and Alden

Preface

Mechanical ventilators can be mysterious and intimidating. When using the ventilator, one is taking on the responsibility of breathing for another human being. Mechanical ventilation is one of the most complex and integral aspects of critical care medicine.

As a pulmonary and critical care physician, I have taught mechanical ventilation to many medical students, residents, and fellows. During these teaching sessions, I have encountered many shared misconceptions about how ventilators work. Much of this misunderstanding stems from the fact that the current nomenclature used in mechanical ventilation is inconsistent and confusing. My hope is that this book clarifies the fundamental concepts of mechanical ventilation.

The ventilator does not function in isolation—it works in concert with the patient's respiratory system. One cannot simply set the ventilator and walk away. Instead, it is important to monitor and adjust the ventilator settings based upon the complex interactions between the ventilator and the patient. Proper ventilator management is not merely a set of prescriptive steps; ventilator settings must be individually and continuously tailored to each patient and unique situation. Therefore, an in-depth understanding of how a ventilator operates is essential to achieving increased patient comfort and optimal patient outcomes.

Learning how to manage patients on ventilators can be daunting. While there are many excellent, comprehensive textbooks on mechanical ventilation, these tomes can be overwhelming to even the most dedicated students. The available "shorter" books are insufficient as they often glance over crucial basic principles. As is the case with learning medicine in general, it is more effective to understand the foundational concepts than to simply memorize algorithms. This book delves into those foundational concepts, and does so clearly and succinctly.

This book is written for anyone who cares for patients requiring mechanical ventilation—physicians, nurses, respiratory therapists—and is intended for providers at all levels of training. It provides the nuts and bolts of how to properly manage the ventilator and serves as a practical resource in the intensive care unit in order to better care for critically ill patients.

New York, NY, USA   Hooman Poor

Contents

Chapter 1
Respiratory Mechanics

Understanding mechanical ventilation must start with a review of the physiology and mechanics of normal spontaneous breathing. **Spontaneous breathing** is defined as movement of air into and out of the lungs as a result of work done by an individual's respiratory muscles. **Positive pressure ventilation**, on the other hand, is defined as movement of air into the lungs by the application of positive pressure to the airway through an endotracheal tube, tracheostomy tube, or noninvasive mask.

Lung Volume

The lungs sit inside a chest cavity surrounded by the chest wall. The potential space between the lungs and the chest wall is known as the **pleural space**. The lungs, composed of elastic tissue, have a tendency to recoil inward, and the chest wall has a tendency to spring outward. If the lungs were removed from the chest cavity and were no longer being influenced by the chest wall or the pleural space, they would collapse like a deflated balloon. Similarly, removing the lungs from the chest cavity would cause the chest wall, no longer being influenced by the lungs or the pleural space, to spring outward. The equilibrium achieved between the lungs' inward recoil and the

© Springer International Publishing AG,
part of Springer Nature 2018
H. Poor, *Basics of Mechanical Ventilation*,
https://doi.org/10.1007/978-3-319-89981-7_1

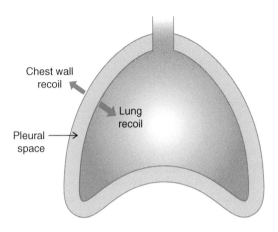

FIGURE 1.1 Chest wall springing outward and lung recoiling inward. Because of these opposing forces, the pleural space has subatmospheric pressure at the end of expiration.

chest wall's outward recoil determines lung volume at the end of expiration. As a result of the coupling of the lungs and the chest wall, pressure in the pleural space, known as **pleural pressure (P_{pl})**, is less than atmospheric pressure at the end of expiration. This subatmospheric pleural pressure prevents the chest wall from springing outward and the lungs from collapsing inward (Fig. 1.1).

> **Key Concept #1**
> Balance between **lung recoil inward** and **chest wall recoil outward** determines lung volume at end of expiration

Transpulmonary Pressure

For a given lung volume at equilibrium, the forces pushing the alveolar walls outward must equal the forces pushing the alveolar walls inward. The expanding outward force is **alveolar**

pressure (P_{alv}). The collapsing inward forces are pleural pressure and **lung elastic recoil pressure (P_{el})**. The difference between alveolar pressure and pleural pressure, known as **transpulmonary pressure (P_{tp})**, is equal and opposite to lung elastic recoil pressure for a given lung volume (Fig. 1.2).

Transpulmonary pressure determines lung volume. Increasing transpulmonary pressure increases the outward distending pressure of the lung, resulting in a larger lung volume. Thus, the lungs can be inflated either by decreasing pleural pressure, as occurs in spontaneous breathing, or by increasing alveolar pressure, as occurs in positive pressure ventilation (Fig. 1.3).

Key Concept #2
- To inflate lungs, P_{tp} must increase
- $P_{tp} = P_{alv} - P_{pl}$
- To increase P_{tp}, either **decrease P_{pl}** (spontaneous breathing) or **increase P_{alv}** (positive pressure ventilation)

The relationship between the transpulmonary pressure and lung volume is not linear, but rather curvilinear, because as lung volume increases, the lungs become stiffer and less compliant. That is, larger increases in transpulmonary pressure are necessary to achieve the same increase in lung volume at higher lung volume than at lower lung volume. Similarly, increasing transpulmonary pressure by a set amount will lead to a larger increase in lung volume at lower lung volume than at higher lung volume (Fig. 1.4).

Spontaneous Breathing

Inspiration

During spontaneous breathing, inspiration occurs by decreasing pleural pressure, which increases transpulmonary pressure

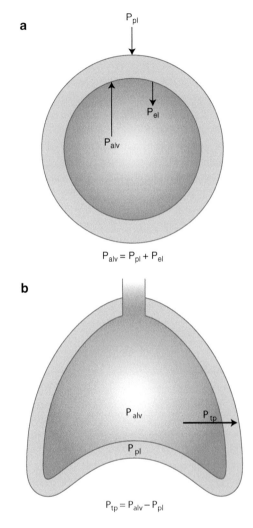

FIGURE 1.2 (**a**) At equilibrium, the sum of the expanding outward forces must equal the sum of the collapsing inward forces at equilibrium. Therefore, alveolar pressure equals the sum of pleural pressure and lung elastic recoil pressure. (**b**) Transpulmonary pressure is the difference between alveolar pressure and pleural pressure. It is equal and opposite to lung elastic recoil pressure for a given lung volume ($P_{tp} = -P_{el}$). P_{alv} alveolar pressure; P_{el} lung elastic recoil pressure; P_{pl} pleural pressure; P_{tp} transpulmonary pressure

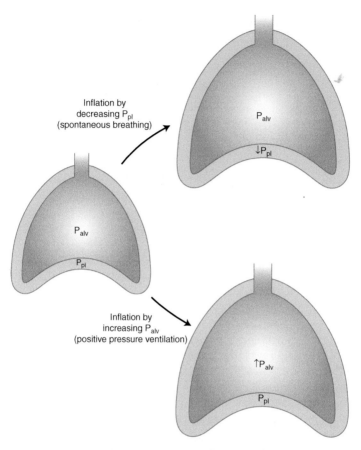

FIGURE 1.3 Lung inflation occurs either by decreasing pleural pressure (spontaneous breathing) or by increasing alveolar pressure (positive pressure ventilation). In both cases, transpulmonary pressure increases.
P_{alv} alveolar pressure; P_{pl} pleural pressure

(remember $P_{tp} = P_{alv} - P_{pl}$). Under normal conditions, alveolar pressure is equal to atmospheric pressure at the end of expiration. During inspiration, the diaphragm and other inspiratory muscles contract, pushing the abdominal contents downward and the rib cage upward and outward, ultimately increasing intrathoracic volume. Boyle's law states that, for a fixed

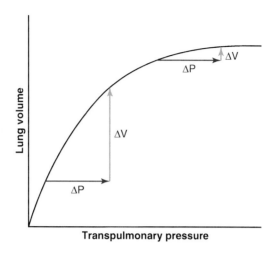

FIGURE 1.4 Relationship between lung volume and transpulmonary pressure. For a given increase in transpulmonary pressure (ΔP), the resultant increase in lung volume (ΔV) is greater at lower lung volume, where the lung is more compliant, than at higher lung volume.

amount of gas kept at constant temperature, pressure and volume are inversely proportional (pressure = 1/volume). Thus, this increase in intrathoracic volume results in a decrease in intrathoracic pressure and therefore a decrease in pleural pressure. Decreased pleural pressure increases transpulmonary pressure and causes the lungs to inflate. This increase in lung volume, as explained by Boyle's law, results in a decrease in alveolar pressure, making it lower than atmospheric pressure. Because gas flows from regions of higher pressure to regions of lower pressure, air flows into the lungs until alveolar pressure equals atmospheric pressure.

Expiration

Quiet expiration is passive. That is, no active contraction of respiratory muscles is required for expiration to occur. The diaphragm and inspiratory muscles relax, the abdominal contents return to their previous position, and the chest wall recoils, ultimately resulting in a decrease in intrathoracic volume. The decrease in intrathoracic volume results in an increase in intrathoracic pressure and thus an increase in pleural pressure. Increased pleural pressure decreases transpulmonary pressure and causes the lungs to deflate. This decrease in lung volume results in an increase in alveolar pressure, making it higher than atmospheric pressure. Because of this pressure gradient, air flows out of the lungs until alveolar pressure equals atmospheric pressure.

Modeling the Respiratory System

The flow of air in and out of the lungs can be modeled in a manner similar to an electrical circuit using Ohm's law, where the voltage (V) across a resistor is equal to the electric current (I) multiplied by the electrical resistance (R). The difference between **proximal airway pressure (P_{air})** measured at the mouth and **alveolar pressure (P_{alv})** is analogous to the voltage difference within a circuit. Similarly, **flow (Q)** and **airway resistance (R)** in the respiratory system are analogous to the electric current and electrical resistance in the circuit, respectively (Fig. 1.5).

The equation for the respiratory system can be rearranged to solve for flow:

$$Q = \frac{P_{air} - P_{alv}}{R}$$

By convention, flow into the patient (inspiration) is designated as positive, and flow out of the patient (expiration) is designated as negative. Note that when proximal airway pressure equals alveolar pressure, there is no flow present in either direction ($Q = 0$). Under normal conditions, this scenario occurs twice during the breathing cycle, at the end of expiration and at the end of inspiration.

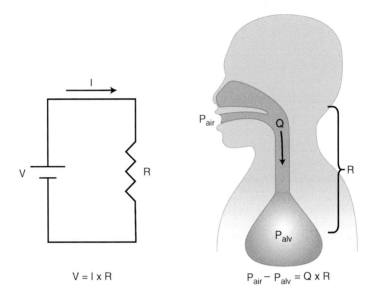

$$V = I \times R$$

$$P_{air} - P_{alv} = Q \times R$$

FIGURE 1.5 The respiratory system modeled as an electrical circuit. I electric current; P_{air} proximal airway pressure; P_{alv} alveolar pressure; Q flow; R resistance; V voltage

With spontaneous breathing, proximal airway pressure is equal to atmospheric pressure. During inspiration, the diaphragm and other inspiratory muscles contract, which increases lung volume and decreases alveolar pressure, as previously discussed. This process results in alveolar pressure being less than proximal airway pressure, which remains at atmospheric pressure. Therefore, flow will become a positive value, indicating that air flows into the patient. During expiration, alveolar pressure is higher than proximal airway pressure, which makes flow a negative value, indicating that air flows out of the patient.

With positive pressure ventilation, as occurs with mechanical ventilation, the ventilator increases proximal airway pressure during inspiration. This increase in proximal airway pressure relative to alveolar pressure results in a positive value for flow, causing air to flow into the patient. Expiration

with positive pressure ventilation is passive and occurs in a
manner similar to that which occurs in spontaneous
breathing.

The sequence of events for inspiration is different for
spontaneous breathing than for positive pressure ventilation.
In spontaneous breathing, increased intrathoracic volume
leads to decreased alveolar pressure, which leads to air flowing into the patient because of the pressure gradient. With
positive pressure ventilation, increased proximal airway pressure leads to air flowing into the patient, which, because of
Boyle's law, results in an increase in lung volume (Fig. 1.6).

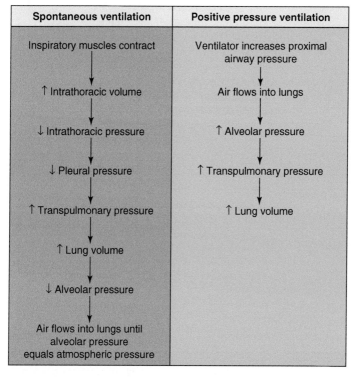

Spontaneous ventilation	Positive pressure ventilation
Inspiratory muscles contract	Ventilator increases proximal airway pressure
↑ Intrathoracic volume	Air flows into lungs
↓ Intrathoracic pressure	↑ Alveolar pressure
↓ Pleural pressure	↑ Transpulmonary pressure
↑ Transpulmonary pressure	↑ Lung volume
↑ Lung volume	
↓ Alveolar pressure	
Air flows into lungs until alveolar pressure equals atmospheric pressure	

FIGURE 1.6 Sequence of events during inspiration for spontaneous
breathing and positive pressure ventilation.

Key Concept #3
- Inspiration with spontaneous breathing: P_{alv} made lower than atmospheric pressure to **suck** air into lungs
- Inspiration with positive pressure ventilation: P_{air} made higher than atmospheric pressure to **push** air into lungs

Suggested Readings

1. Cairo J. Pilbeam's mechanical ventilation: physiological and clinical applications. 5th ed. St. Louis: Mosby; 2012.
2. Costanzo L. Physiology. 5th ed. Beijing: Saunders; 2014.
3. Rhoades R, Bell D. Medical physiology: principles for clinical medicine. 4th ed. Philadelphia: Lippincott Williams & Wilkins; 2013.
4. Broaddus V, Ernst J. Murray and Nadel's textbook of respiratory medicine. 5th ed. Philadelphia: Saunders; 2010.
5. West J. Respiratory physiology: the essentials. 9th ed. Philadelphia: Lippincott Williams & Wilkins; 2012.

Chapter 2
Phase Variables

A ventilator is a machine that delivers a flow of gas for a certain amount of time by increasing proximal airway pressure, a process which culminates in a delivered tidal volume. Because of the imprecise, inconsistent, and outdated terminology used to describe modern ventilators, many clinicians often misunderstand exactly how a ventilator functions. Understanding the exact instructions that a ventilator follows to deliver a breath for the various modes of ventilation is crucial for optimal ventilator management.

Anatomy of a Breath

Breathing is a periodic event, composed of repeated cycles of inspiration and expiration. Each breath, defined as one cycle of inspiration followed by expiration, can be broken down into four components, known as **phase variables**. These phase variables determine when inspiration begins (**trigger**), how flow is delivered during inspiration (**target**), when inspiration ends (**cycle**), and proximal airway pressure during expiration (**baseline**) (Fig. 2.1).

© Springer International Publishing AG, part of Springer Nature 2018
H. Poor, *Basics of Mechanical Ventilation*, https://doi.org/10.1007/978-3-319-89981-7_2

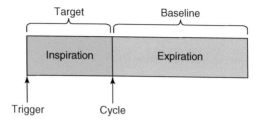

FIGURE 2.1 Schematic of a breath cycle. The trigger variable determines when expiration ends and inspiration begins. The cycle variable determines when inspiration ends and expiration begins. The target variable determines flow during inspiration. The baseline variable determines proximal airway pressure during expiration.

Key Concept #1
Ventilator phase variables:

- Trigger: when inspiration begins
- Target: how flow is delivered during inspiration
- Cycle: when inspiration ends
- Baseline: proximal airway pressure during expiration

Trigger

The trigger variable determines when to initiate inspiration. Breaths can either be **ventilator-triggered** or **patient-triggered**. Ventilator-triggered breaths use time as the trigger variable. Patient-triggered breaths are initiated by patient respiratory efforts, utilizing pressure or flow for the trigger variable.

Time Trigger

With time triggering, the ventilator initiates a breath after a set amount of time has elapsed since the initiation of the previous breath. The most common manner to set the time trigger is by setting the respiratory rate (time = 1/rate). For example, setting the ventilator respiratory rate to 12 breaths per minute is equivalent to setting the time trigger to 5 seconds because one breath every 5 seconds will result in 12 breaths per minute. When a breath is initiated by a time trigger, that breath is classified as a ventilator-triggered, or **control**, breath.

Key Concept #2
- **Control** breath = **ventilator**-triggered breath
- Trigger variable for control breath = **time**

Patient Trigger

Changes in pressure and flow in the circuit as a result of patient respiratory efforts are detected by the ventilator. When the patient makes an inspiratory effort, as discussed in Chap. 1, the diaphragm and inspiratory muscles contract, lowering pleural pressure, which ultimately reduces proximal airway pressure. This reduced airway pressure is transmitted along the ventilator tubing and measured by the ventilator. If a pressure trigger is set and the magnitude of the reduction in proximal airway pressure as measured by the ventilator is greater than the set pressure trigger, a breath will be initiated and delivered by the ventilator (Fig. 2.2).

For flow-triggering, a continuous amount of gas flows from the inspiratory limb of the ventilator to the expiratory limb of the ventilator during the expiratory (baseline) phase. This flow is continuously measured by the ventilator. In the absence of any patient inspiratory efforts, the flow of gas leaving the ventilator through the inspiratory limb should equal the flow of gas returning to the ventilator through the expiratory limb. During a patient inspiratory effort, some of this flow will enter the patient instead of returning to the ventilator, and the ventilator will detect decreased flow into the expiratory limb. If this reduction in flow returning to the ventilator exceeds the set flow trigger, a breath will be initiated and delivered by the ventilator (Fig. 2.3).

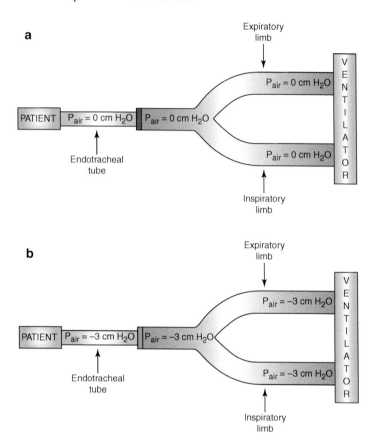

FIGURE 2.2 Respiratory circuit demonstrating the pressure trigger mechanism. (a) Assuming that no external positive end-expiratory pressure is added, pressure in the respiratory circuit at baseline is 0 cm H_2O. (b) A patient's inspiratory effort will cause a decrease in the patient's proximal airway pressure, leading to a decrease in airway pressure of the respiratory circuit, which can be detected by the ventilator. In this example, pressure in the respiratory circuit has decreased by 3 cm H_2O. If the pressure trigger threshold is set at 3 cm H_2O or less, this inspiratory effort would trigger the ventilator to deliver a breath.

P_{air} proximal airway pressure

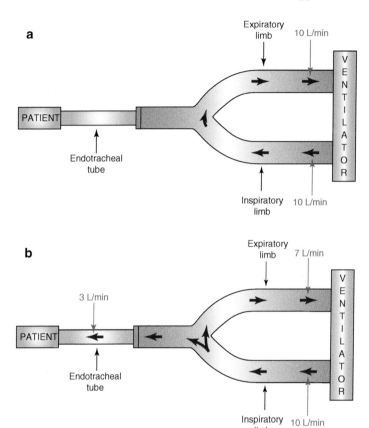

FIGURE 2.3 Respiratory circuit demonstrating the flow trigger mechanism. (**a**) A continuous amount of gas flows from the inspiratory limb to the expiratory limb of the ventilator. In this example, the continuous gas flow is 10 L/min. (**b**) A patient's inspiratory effort will cause some of the flow to enter the patient instead of returning to the ventilator. In this example, 3 L/min of flow is entering the patient, resulting in 3 L/min less flow returning to the ventilator. If the flow trigger threshold is set at 3 L/min or less, this inspiratory effort would trigger the ventilator to deliver a breath.

When a breath is initiated by a pressure or flow trigger, that breath is classified as a patient-triggered, or **assist**, breath. The difference between pressure and flow triggers in modern ventilators is generally clinically insignificant. A patient can trigger the ventilator only during the expiratory (baseline) phase. Patient respiratory efforts during inspiration after a breath has been initiated will not trigger another breath.

> **Key Concept #3**
> - **Assist** breath = **patient**-triggered breath
> - Trigger variable for assist breath = **pressure** or **flow**

Assist-Control

A patient trigger (assist) and a ventilator trigger (control) can be combined to create a hybrid trigger mode known as **assist-control (A/C)**. With this hybrid trigger, both a control respiratory rate (time trigger) and either a pressure or flow trigger are set. If an amount of time as set by the time trigger has elapsed without a patient-triggered breath, the ventilator will initiate a "control" breath. However, if the patient triggers the ventilator, via the pressure or flow trigger, prior to elapsing of the time trigger, the ventilator will initiate an "assist" breath and the time trigger clock will reset. It is important to note that there are no differences in the other characteristics of a breath (i.e., target, cycle, and baseline) between a time-triggered "control" breath and a patient-triggered "assist" breath. "Assist" and "control" only describe whether the breath was triggered by the patient or by the ventilator, respectively.

> **Key Concept #4**
> - **A/C** combines two triggers: patient trigger (**assist**) and ventilator trigger (**control**)
> - **A/C** refers *only* to the trigger, not to other phase variables

Many ventilators indicate whether the delivered breath was a "control" or "assist" breath, often with a flashing "A" or "C" on the display. Additionally, one can determine whether a delivered breath was a "control" or "assist" breath by examining the pressure curve on the ventilator screen. Patient-triggered "assist" breaths will have a negative deflection on the pressure curve right before inspiration, whereas time-triggered "control" breaths will not. A downward deflection of the pressure tracing for patient-triggered breaths is reflective of the patient inspiratory effort, resulting in a reduction in proximal airway pressure (Fig. 2.4).

The actual respiratory rate of the ventilator will depend on the relationship between the time-triggered control rate and the rate of inspiratory effort by the patient. Assuming the intrinsic breathing pattern of the patient is regular, if the time trigger is set such that the control rate is 10 breaths per minute (one breath every 6 seconds), and the rate of patient inspiratory efforts is 20 breaths per minute (one breath every 3 seconds), then all of the breaths will be "assist" breaths because the patient will trigger the ventilator prior to the

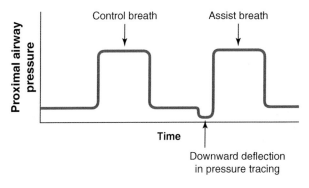

FIGURE 2.4 Pressure tracing demonstrating a ventilator-triggered "control" breath and a patient-triggered "assist" breath. Proximal airway pressure is plotted on the vertical (y) axis, and time is plotted on the horizontal (x) axis. Note the downward deflection in the pressure tracing prior to the assist breath, indicating that a patient inspiratory effort triggered the ventilator.

time trigger elapsing. Therefore, the actual respiratory rate will be 20 breaths per minute. In this case, increasing the control respiratory rate on the ventilator from 10 to 15 breaths per minute (reducing the time trigger from 6 to 4 seconds) will have no effect on the respiratory rate if the patient continues to trigger the ventilator every 3 seconds. However, increasing the set respiratory rate to above 20 breaths per minute (decreasing the time trigger to below 3 seconds) will result in all of the breaths being time-triggered control breaths. The set time-triggered respiratory rate is essentially a "backup" rate—if the patient does not trigger the ventilator at a frequency higher than the backup rate, the ventilator will deliver time-triggered control breaths at the set backup respiratory rate.

Most ventilators display the actual respiratory rate. If the actual respiratory rate is higher than the time-triggered "control" respiratory rate, there must be patient-triggered "assist" breaths present. For patients with irregular breathing patterns where the time between patient inspiratory efforts varies, there can be a combination of patient-triggered "assist" breaths and time-triggered "control" breaths.

Target

The target variable is probably the most misunderstood of the phase variables. Part of this confusion arises from the fact that other names are commonly used for this variable, including "control" and "limit."

The target variable regulates how flow is administered *during* inspiration. The variables most commonly used for the target include flow and pressure. Volume, specifically tidal volume, is technically not a target variable because it does not clarify how the flow is to be delivered—setting a tidal volume does not determine whether that volume is to be delivered over a short period of time (high flow rate) or a long period of time (low flow rate). Note that volume delivered *per unit time*, which is the definition of flow, is a target variable.

Key Concept #5
- Target variable can be **flow** or **pressure**
- **Volume** is not a target variable (but can be a cycle variable)

The equation from Chap. 1 relating flow, pressure, and resistance of the respiratory system helps elucidate the role of the target variable:

$$Q = \frac{P_{air} - P_{alv}}{R}$$

Q = flow
P_{air} = proximal airway pressure
P_{alv} = alveolar pressure
R = airway resistance

The target variable is the independent variable in this equation, its value set by the provider and dutifully achieved by the ventilator. The target can be either flow or proximal airway pressure, but not both at the same time. When either flow or proximal airway pressure is set by the ventilator as the target variable, the other variable becomes a dependent variable, its value determined by the target variable, resistance, and alveolar pressure.

Flow Target

With a flow target, flow is selected as the independent variable. The ventilator simply delivers the flow as set by the provider. Therefore, proximal airway pressure becomes dependent on flow (target variable), resistance, and alveolar pressure. The flow waveform pattern, which describes the pattern of gas flow, is also selected. The most commonly used flow waveforms are constant flow and decelerating ramp.

With the constant flow waveform pattern, also known as the square or rectangle waveform pattern, the inspiratory flow rate instantly rises to the set level and remains constant during the inspiratory cycle. With the decelerating ramp waveform pattern, the inspiratory flow rate is highest at the beginning of inspiration, when patient flow demand is often greatest, and then depreciates to zero flow (Fig. 2.5).

Pressure Target

With a pressure target, the proximal airway pressure is selected as the independent variable. The ventilator delivers flow to quickly achieve and maintain proximal airway pressure during inspiration. Therefore, flow becomes dependent on proximal airway pressure (target variable), resistance, and alveolar pressure (Fig. 2.6).

Pressure-targeted modes naturally produce a decelerating ramp flow waveform. The prior equation can be used to elucidate why:

$$Q = \frac{P_{air} - P_{alv}}{R}$$

During the inspiratory phase, as air fills the alveoli, alveolar pressure increases. Since proximal airway pressure remains constant during the inspiratory phase of a pressure-targeted breath, and assuming resistance does not significantly change during the breath, flow must decrease as alveolar pressure increases. Therefore, flow will be highest at the beginning of the breath and decrease as the inspiratory phase proceeds.

Key Concept #6
- Pressure-targeted modes produce decelerating ramp flow waveforms

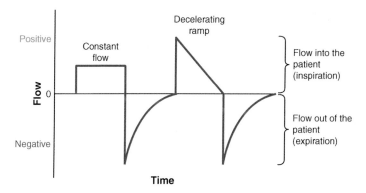

FIGURE 2.5 Constant flow and decelerating ramp waveform patterns. Flow is plotted on the vertical (y) axis, and time is plotted on the horizontal (x) axis. Flow going into the patient (inspiration) is denoted as positive flow, while flow coming out of the patient (expiration) is denoted as negative flow.

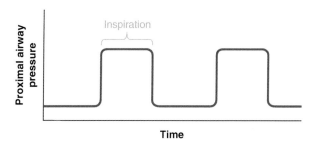

FIGURE 2.6 Pressure waveform. Proximal airway pressure is plotted on the vertical (y) axis, and time is plotted on the horizontal (x) axis. Note that proximal airway pressure is constant during inspiration.

Flow Vs. Pressure Target

The difference between modes using flow and pressure targets is most evident when there is a change in the respiratory system, either because of a change in resistance or compliance or as a result of patient respiratory efforts. When a change in the respiratory system occurs, the set target variable remains unchanged, while the other, dependent variable changes, as the ventilator cannot set both flow and proximal airway pressure simultaneously.

To illustrate this difference, imagine two patients, Patient A and Patient B, with identical respiratory systems receiving mechanical ventilation (Fig. 2.7). Patient A has a flow-targeted mode, while Patient B has a pressure-targeted mode. If the two patients bite their endotracheal tubes during the inspiratory phase, each patient will experience an acute rise in airway resistance. In this scenario, the two ventilator modes will respond differently to the change in the respiratory system. For Patient A, since the target variable is flow, flow remains unaffected, and higher proximal airway pressure is required to maintain the set flow. For Patient B, since the target variable is pressure, proximal airway pressure remains unaffected, and lower flow is required to maintain the set proximal airway pressure.

If, instead of biting the endotracheal tubes, the patients make a sustained respiratory effort by contracting their inspiratory muscles during inspiration, each patient will experience a decrease in alveolar pressure. In this scenario, the two ventilator modes will again respond differently to the change in the respiratory system. For Patient A, since the target variable is flow, flow remains unaffected, and lower proximal airway pressure is required to maintain the set flow. For Patient B, since the target variable is pressure, proximal airway pressure remains unaffected, and higher flow is required to maintain the set proximal airway pressure.

Key Concept #7
- Flow and proximal airway pressure cannot be set as the target simultaneously
- When one variable is set as the target, the other will vary with changes in the respiratory system

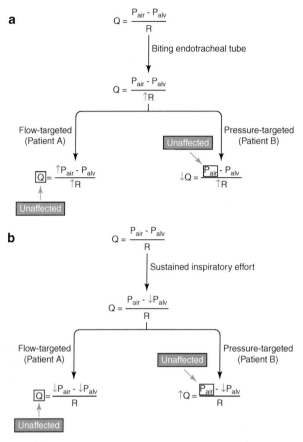

FIGURE 2.7 Flow chart demonstrating the response of flow-targeted and pressure-targeted modes to changes in the respiratory system. (**a**) Biting of the endotracheal tube increases airway resistance. In flow-targeted modes, because flow is set, it remains unaffected, and therefore proximal airway pressure increases. In pressure-targeted modes, because proximal airway pressure is set, it remains unaffected, and therefore flow decreases. (**b**) Sustained inspiratory effort by the patient reduces pleural pressure, which reduces alveolar pressure. In flow-targeted modes, because flow is set, it remains unaffected, and therefore proximal airway pressure decreases. In pressure-targeted modes, because proximal airway pressure is set, it remains unaffected, and therefore flow increases.

P_{air} proximal airway pressure; P_{alv} alveolar pressure; Q flow; R resistance

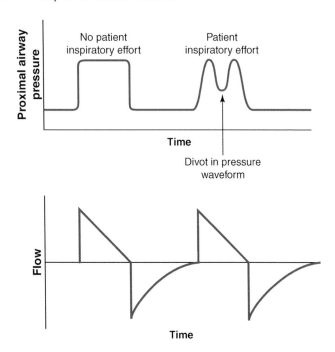

FIGURE 2.8 Flow and pressure waveforms of a flow-targeted mode demonstrating the response to a sustained patient inspiratory effort. A patient inspiratory effort, which decreases alveolar pressure, will not affect the flow waveform because the flow waveform is set in a flow-targeted mode. Instead, there will be a decrease in proximal airway pressure during the inspiratory effort, as represented by a divot in the pressure waveform.

Significant inspiratory efforts by a patient can be detected in those receiving flow-targeted ventilation by examining the pressure waveform. Because proximal airway pressure decreases with inspiratory efforts, divots in the pressure waveform during a flow-targeted mode are indicative of patient inspiratory efforts (Fig. 2.8). It is important to note that a patient, despite making inspiratory efforts that reduce airway pressure, cannot trigger the ventilator during the inspiratory phase. The patient can only trigger the ventilator during the expiratory (baseline) phase.

Key Concept #8
- In a flow-targeted mode, divots in the pressure waveform indicate patient inspiratory efforts

Cycle

The cycle variable determines when to terminate the inspiratory phase of a breath. The term "to cycle" is synonymous with "to terminate inspiration." The variables most commonly used for the cycle include volume, time, and flow.

For volume-cycled breaths, the inspiratory phase continues until a set volume has been delivered. For time-cycled breaths, the inspiratory phase continues until a set time has elapsed. For flow-cycled breaths, the inspiratory phase continues until the inspiratory flow diminishes to a set value. Flow-cycling is most commonly utilized with pressure-targeted modes, where flow is delivered to maintain a specified airway pressure. As mentioned above, pressure-targeted modes naturally produce a decelerating ramp flow waveform, with flow highest at the beginning of the breath and decreasing as the inspiratory phase proceeds. With flow-cycling, the ventilator is set to terminate the breath when the inspiratory flow diminishes to a selected percentage of the peak inspiratory flow. Increasing the percentage of the peak inspiratory flow for cycling to occur decreases the inspiratory time and vice versa (Fig. 2.9).

Pressure-cycling is not commonly used as an exclusive cycling modality but is often employed in conjunction with flow-targeted, volume-cycled modes as a safety mechanism to prevent the generation of dangerously high airway pressures. If excessively high airway pressures are reached before the set tidal volume has been delivered, the pressure-cycling mechanism will terminate inspiration.

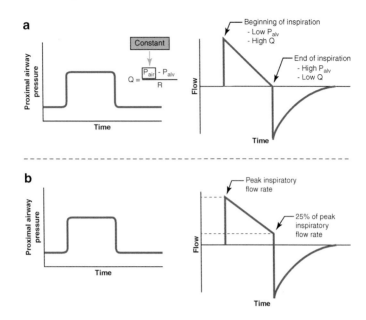

FIGURE 2.9 (**a**) Pressure and flow waveforms in a pressure-targeted mode demonstrating a decelerating ramp flow waveform. With pressure-targeted modes, proximal airway pressure is constant during the inspiratory phase. As air fills the alveoli, alveolar pressure increases. Assuming resistance does not significantly change, flow decreases as inspiration progresses, producing a decelerating ramp flow waveform. (**b**) Pressure and flow waveforms in a pressure-targeted, flow-cycled mode. With a pressure-targeted mode, inspiratory flow is highest at the beginning of inspiration, depreciating as inspiration continues. With flow-cycling, the breath terminates once flow depreciates to a set percentage of the peak inspiratory flow, in this case 25%.
P_{air} proximal airway pressure; P_{alv} alveolar pressure; Q flow; R resistance

Baseline

The baseline variable refers to the proximal airway pressure during the expiratory phase. This pressure can be equal to atmospheric pressure, known as zero end-expiratory pressure (ZEEP), in which the ventilator allows for complete recoil of

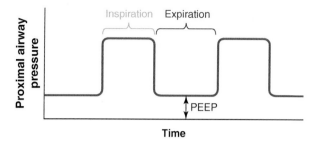

Figure 2.10 Pressure waveform demonstrating positive end-expiratory pressure.
PEEP positive end-expiratory pressure

the lung and chest wall, or it can be held above atmospheric pressure by the ventilator, known as positive end-expiratory pressure (PEEP) (Fig. 2.10). The utility of PEEP will be discussed in Chap. 5 (Acute Respiratory Distress Syndrome) and Chap. 6 (Obstructive Lung Diseases).

In the next chapter, these phase variables will be mixed and matched to construct the common modes of ventilation.

Suggested Readings

1. Cairo J. Pilbeam's mechanical ventilation: physiological and clinical applications. 5th ed. St. Louis: Mosby; 2012.
2. Chatburn R. Classification of ventilator modes: update and proposal for implementation. Respir Care. 2007;52:301–23.
3. Chatburn R, El-Khatib M, Mireles-Cabodevila E. A taxonomy for mechanical ventilation: 10 fundamental maxims. Respir Care. 2014;59:1747–63.
4. MacIntyre N. Design features of modern mechanical ventilators. Clin Chest Med. 2016;37:607–13.
5. MacIntyre N, Branson R. Mechanical ventilation. 2nd ed. Philadelphia: Saunders; 2009.
6. Tobin M. Principles and practice of mechanical ventilation. 3rd ed. Beijing: McGraw-Hill; 2013.

Chapter 3
Basic Modes of Ventilation

Each mode of ventilation is defined by its phase variable components: trigger, target, and cycle. These phase variables are explained in detail in Chap. 2. The three basic modes of ventilation include **volume-controlled ventilation (VCV), pressure-controlled ventilation (PCV),** and **pressure support ventilation (PSV)**.

Volume-Controlled Ventilation

The trigger variable for VCV is assist-control, a hybrid between a patient trigger and a ventilator trigger. The patient-triggered (assist) component of the trigger can utilize either a pressure or flow trigger. The ventilator-triggered (control) component of the trigger is set by selecting the respiratory rate, which dictates the time between control breaths (rate = 1/time).

The target variable is flow. Both the flow rate and the flow waveform pattern are selected on the ventilator. The most commonly used flow waveform patterns are the constant flow and the decelerating ramp.

The cycle variable is volume. Tidal volume is selected on the ventilator. Because flow is set, setting tidal volume will also determine inspiratory time (time = volume/flow);

© Springer International Publishing AG, 29
part of Springer Nature 2018
H. Poor, *Basics of Mechanical Ventilation*,
https://doi.org/10.1007/978-3-319-89981-7_3

therefore, inspiratory time cannot be altered by patient respiratory effort or by changes in the respiratory system.

In summary, VCV is a flow-targeted, volume-cycled mode of ventilation in which the ventilator delivers a set flow waveform pattern to achieve a set tidal volume. The pressure waveform will vary depending on characteristics of the respiratory system and patient respiratory effort (Fig. 3.1 and Table 3.1).

> **Key Concept #1**
> VCV = **flow**-targeted, **volume**-cycled

Pressure-Controlled Ventilation

The trigger variable for PCV is assist-control, exactly the same as VCV. The target variable is pressure. Proximal airway pressure is selected on the ventilator. Flow is delivered by the ventilator to quickly achieve and maintain the set proximal airway pressure. As described in Chap. 2, a constant airway pressure during inspiration produces a decelerating ramp flow waveform.

The cycle variable is time. The inspiratory time is selected on the ventilator. Inspiration will end after the set inspiratory time has elapsed. Similar to VCV, inspiratory time cannot be altered by patient respiratory effort or by changes in the respiratory system.

FIGURE 3.1 Flow and pressure waveforms in VCV. The target variable for VCV is flow. Both decelerating ramp (**a**) and constant flow (**b**) waveforms are demonstrated. The cycle variable for VCV is volume, which equals the area under the flow waveform curve (shaded region). The inspiratory flow waveform is set by the clinician. The pressure waveform is a result of the interaction between the set variables (flow-targeted and volume-cycled) and the respiratory system. *VCV* volume-controlled ventilation

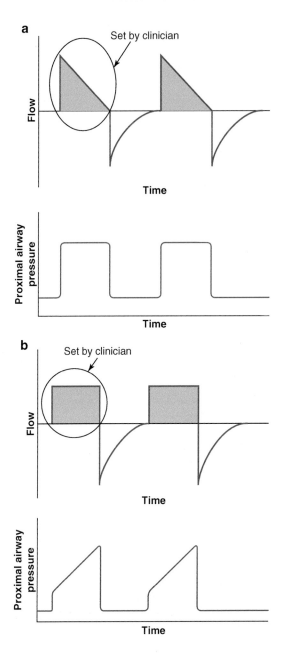

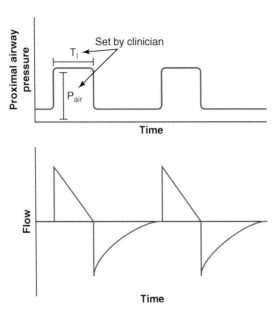

FIGURE 3.2 Flow and pressure waveforms in PCV. The target variable for PCV is pressure. The cycle variable for PCV is time. Proximal airway pressure and inspiratory time are set by the clinician. The flow waveform is a result of the interaction between the set variables (pressure-targeted and time-cycled) and the respiratory system. The resultant flow waveform in PCV is a decelerating ramp. P_{air} proximal airway pressure; *PCV* pressure-controlled ventilation; T_I inspiratory time

In summary, PCV is a pressure-targeted, time-cycled mode of ventilation, in which the ventilator delivers flow to quickly achieve and maintain a set proximal airway pressure for a set amount of time. The flow waveform will vary depending on characteristics of the respiratory system and patient respiratory effort (Fig. 3.2 and Table 3.1).

Key Concept #2
PCV = **pressure**-targeted, **time**-cycled

Pressure Support Ventilation

The trigger variable for PSV consists of only the patient (assist) trigger. As with the assist component of the assist-control trigger for both VCV and PCV, the trigger can be set as either a flow or a pressure trigger. There are no time-triggered, control breaths; therefore, this mode of ventilation can only be used if the patient initiates a sufficient number of breaths per minute.

The target variable is pressure. Just like with PCV, proximal airway pressure is selected on the ventilator. Flow is delivered by the ventilator to quickly achieve and maintain the set proximal airway pressure. The constant airway pressure during inspiration produces a decelerating ramp flow waveform, similar to that seen with PCV.

The cycle variable is flow. The ventilator is set to terminate the breath once flow diminishes to a specified percentage of peak inspiratory flow (e.g., 25%). This cycling mechanism utilizes the fact that a constant proximal airway pressure during inspiration produces a decelerating ramp flow waveform, in which flow is highest at the beginning of the breath and then decreases as the inspiratory phase proceeds.

While the inspiratory time in VCV and PCV is predetermined and does not change from breath to breath, the inspiratory time in PSV can vary. Inspiratory time in PSV is not constrained because breath cycling in this mode depends on the depreciation of flow. Flow in pressure-targeted modes, as discussed in Chap. 2, varies with changes in respiratory system resistance and compliance, as well as patient respiratory effort. Thus, patients can regulate inspiratory time with PSV by adjusting their respiratory effort, resulting in greater patient comfort and less patient-ventilator dyssynchrony.

In summary, PSV is a pressure-targeted, flow-cycled mode of ventilation, in which the ventilator delivers flow to quickly achieve and maintain a set airway pressure until the inspiratory flow depreciates to a set percentage of peak inspiratory flow. The flow waveform, tidal volume, and inspiratory time vary depending on characteristics of the respiratory system and patient respiratory effort (Fig. 3.3 and Table 3.1).

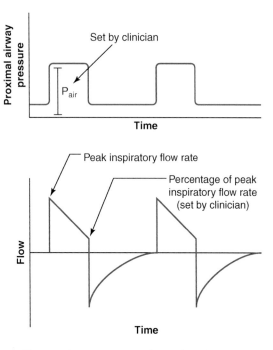

FIGURE 3.3 Flow and pressure waveforms in PSV. The target variable for PSV is pressure. The cycle variable for PSV is flow. Proximal airway pressure and the percentage of peak inspiratory flow for cycling are set by the clinician. The flow waveform is a result of the interaction between the set variables (pressure-targeted and flow-cycled) and the respiratory system. Similar to PCV, the resultant flow waveform in PSV is a decelerating ramp. With flow-cycling, the breath terminates once flow depreciates to a set percentage of the peak flow, in this case 25%.

P_{air} proximal airway pressure; *PSV* pressure support ventilation

Key Concept #3
PSV = **pressure**-targeted, **flow**-cycled

Key Concept #4
- VCV and PCV use **A/C** trigger
- PSV uses only patient **assist** trigger

TABLE 3.1 Summary of the basic modes of ventilation

Mode of ventilation	Trigger	Target	Cycle
VCV	Assist-control	Flow	Volume
PCV	Assist-control	Pressure	Time
PSV	Assist	Pressure	Flow

Volume-Controlled Ventilation Vs. Pressure-Controlled Ventilation

VCV and PCV are similar in that they both use assist-control as the trigger. Additionally, both modes of ventilation have a predetermined inspiratory time, which cannot be altered by patient effort or by changes in the respiratory system. In PCV, the inspiratory time is directly set, whereas in VCV, inspiratory time is determined by setting flow (target) and tidal volume (cycle).

Key Concept #5
- VCV and PCV: inspiratory time cannot vary from breath to breath
- PSV: inspiratory time can vary from breath to breath

It is important to note that in both modes of ventilation, a flow waveform is delivered, resulting in a pressure waveform, and culminating in a delivered tidal volume. In VCV, flow and volume are set, producing a resultant proximal airway pressure. In PCV, proximal airway pressure and inspiratory time are set, producing a resultant flow and volume. If the respiratory system (resistance and compliance) remains unchanged, switching between these modes of ventilation would not result in changes to the ventilator output.

Imagine a patient receiving PCV with proximal airway pressure (target) set to 20 cm H_2O and inspiratory time (cycle) set to 1 second. Now imagine that the respiratory system is such that these PCV settings result in a decelerating ramp flow waveform with peak flow of 60 L/minute and tidal volume of 500 mL. If this same patient were switched from PCV to VCV with a decelerating ramp flow waveform (target), peak flow set to 60 L/minute (target), and tidal volume set to 500 mL (cycle), the resultant proximal airway pressure would be 20 cm H_2O, and the resultant inspiratory time would be 1 second, which were the previous PCV settings. Given that the characteristics of the respiratory system have remained unchanged, flow, tidal volume, proximal airway pressure, and inspiratory time are the same in both cases (Fig. 3.4).

What distinguishes these two modes of ventilation is the response to changes in the respiratory system, either because of a change in resistance or compliance, or as a result of patient respiratory efforts. As explained in Chap. 2, the target and cycle variables remain unchanged, while the other variables change. If a patient is receiving VCV and bites the endotracheal tube, causing an increase in airway resistance, flow (target) and volume (cycle) remain unchanged, while airway pressure increases. Alternatively, if a patient is receiving PCV and bites the endotracheal tube, proximal airway pressure (target) and inspiratory time (cycle) remain unchanged, while flow, and consequently volume, decrease. If a patient is receiving VCV and makes a sustained inspiratory effort during inspiration, flow (target) and volume (cycle) remain unchanged, while proximal airway pressure decreases. Alternatively, if a patient is receiving PCV and makes a sustained inspiratory effort during inspiration, proximal airway pressure (target) and inspiratory time (cycle) remain unchanged, while flow, and consequently volume, increase.

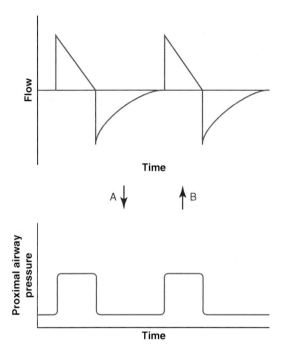

FIGURE 3.4 Flow and pressure waveforms. For a given resistance and compliance of the respiratory system, setting a flow waveform (as occurs with volume-controlled ventilation) will result in a distinct pressure waveform (**A**). If the respiratory system does not change, setting that same pressure waveform (as occurs with pressure-controlled ventilation) will result in the original flow waveform (**B**).

Pressure-Controlled Ventilation Vs. Pressure Support Ventilation

PCV and PSV are both pressure-targeted modes. That is, during the inspiratory phase for each mode, flow is delivered to achieve and maintain a set pressure. The only differences between the two modes of ventilation are during the trigger and cycle phases.

The trigger for PCV is assist-control, a hybrid of a patient trigger (assist) and a ventilator trigger (control). The trigger for PSV, on the other hand, consists only of a patient trigger and lacks the ventilator trigger. The patient trigger for both PCV and PSV are the same and can be set by either using a pressure or a flow trigger. Therefore, a patient receiving PCV who is triggering the ventilator at a rate faster than the set control rate, such that all of the breaths are "assist," will have absolutely no change in the triggering mechanism if the mode were switched to PSV.

The cycle for PCV is time, which does not vary from breath to breath and cannot be altered by patient effort or by changes in the respiratory system. The cycle for PSV is flow, specifically a percentage of the peak inspiratory flow rate. In contrast to PCV, inspiratory time in PSV can vary with changes in respiratory system resistance and compliance, as well as with patient respiratory effort.

Suggested Readings

1. Cairo J. Pilbeam's mechanical ventilation: physiological and clinical applications. 5th ed. St. Louis: Mosby; 2012.
2. Chatburn R. Classification of ventilator modes: update and proposal for implementation. Respir Care. 2007;52:301–23.
3. Chatburn R, El-Khatib M, Mireles-Cabodevila E. A taxonomy for mechanical ventilation: 10 fundamental maxims. Respir Care. 2014;59:1747–63.
4. MacIntyre N. Design features of modern mechanical ventilators. Clin Chest Med. 2016;37:607–13.
5. MacIntyre N, Branson R. Mechanical ventilation. 2nd ed. Philadelphia: Saunders; 2009.
6. Rittayamai N, Katsios C, Beloncle F, et al. Pressure-controlled vs volume-controlled ventilation in acute respiratory failure: a physiology-based narrative and systemic review. Chest. 2015;148:340–55.
7. Tobin M. Principles and practice of mechanical ventilation. 3rd ed. Beijing: McGraw-Hill; 2013.

Chapter 4
Monitoring Respiratory Mechanics

Not only does the ventilator act therapeutically to support ventilation and gas exchange; it can also provide critical information regarding a patient's respiratory mechanics, which can aid in the diagnosis of the patient's respiratory failure.

Two-Component Model

To understand how the ventilator provides information about respiratory mechanics, it is helpful to break down the respiratory system into two components: the **resistive component** and the **elastic component**. The resistive component is determined by the airways, which are comprised of the endotracheal tube and the patient's own airways. The elastic component is determined by the lung parenchyma and the chest wall. **Elastance**, the inverse of compliance, is a measure of stiffness. The ventilator must provide adequate airway pressure to push air through the resistive component (creating flow), an action analogous to blowing air through a tube. The ventilator must also provide adequate airway pressure to inflate the elastic component (filling with volume), an action analogous to inflating a balloon. Therefore, proximal airway

© Springer International Publishing AG,
part of Springer Nature 2018
H. Poor, *Basics of Mechanical Ventilation*,
https://doi.org/10.1007/978-3-319-89981-7_4

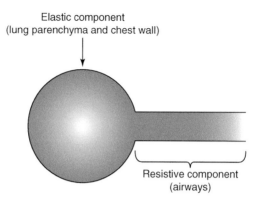

Elastic component
(lung parenchyma and chest wall)

Resistive component
(airways)

$P_{air} = P_R + P_E$

FIGURE 4.1 Two-component model of the respiratory system. The respiratory system is composed of a resistive component (airways) and an elastic component (lung parenchyma and chest wall). P_{air} proximal airway pressure; P_E elastic component of proximal airway pressure; P_R resistive component of proximal airway pressure

pressure is equal to the sum of pressure arising from the resistive component and pressure arising from the elastic component (Fig. 4.1).

> **Key Concept #1**
> Two-component model of the respiratory system:
>
> • Resistive component = airways
> • Elastic component = lung parenchyma and chest wall

The resistive component of proximal airway pressure (P_R) is equal to the product of flow (Q) and resistance (R), a relationship analogous to Ohm's law, as described in Chap. 1. Increasing either flow through the tube or increasing resistance of the tube will increase airway pressure:

$$P_R = Q \times R$$

The elastic component of proximal airway pressure (P_E) is equal to volume (V) in the lungs divided by compliance (C)

of the respiratory system. Increasing tidal volume or decreasing compliance (increasing stiffness) will increase airway pressure:

$$P_E = \frac{V}{C}$$

Putting these two components together provides the equation for proximal airway pressure:

$$P_{air} = Q \times R + \frac{V}{C}$$

Note that this equation is merely a rearrangement of the equation from Chap. 1 (P_{alv} = alveolar pressure):

$$Q = \frac{P_{air} - P_{alv}}{R}$$

V/C is substituted for P_{alv}:

$$Q = \frac{P_{air} - \dfrac{V}{C}}{R}$$

The equation is rearranged:

$$P_{air} = Q \times R + \frac{V}{C}$$

Key Concept #2
- Compliance is a measure of "stretchiness"
- Elastance is a measure of "stiffness"
- Compliance is the reciprocal of elastance

Airway Pressures

Ventilators have pressure gauges that continuously report proximal airway pressure during mechanical ventilation. Evaluating this proximal airway pressure relative to flow and tidal volume can provide information about a patient's respiratory mechanics, specifically resistance and compliance of the respiratory system.

In the setting of volume-controlled ventilation (VCV), flow (target) and tidal volume (cycle) are set. Therefore, proximal airway pressure will depend on resistance of the airways and compliance of the lung parenchyma and chest wall. **Peak airway pressure** is the maximum proximal airway pressure during the respiratory cycle. For a given flow rate and tidal volume, peak airway pressure will be elevated in the setting of increased resistance or decreased compliance. In order to determine whether increased peak airway pressure is a result of increased resistance or decreased compliance, an **inspiratory pause maneuver** can be performed. With this maneuver, after the set tidal volume is delivered, the expiratory valve of the ventilator closes, preventing air from leaving the respiratory system for a short period of time. Because air cannot leave the respiratory system during this time period, pressure everywhere in the respiratory system equalizes. When pressure across the entire respiratory system has equalized, there is no longer any pressure gradient to drive flow, so flow ceases ($Q = 0$). As noted, $P_R = Q \times R$, and therefore P_R (the resistive component of proximal airway pressure) will also be zero, regardless of airway resistance. Thus, the measured proximal airway pressure consists only of that which arises from the elastic component (P_E), which is equal to V/C.

Proximal airway pressure measured at the end of the inspiratory pause maneuver is known as **plateau pressure**. Plateau pressure will increase with increased tidal volume or decreased respiratory system compliance. Plateau pressure can be viewed as the maximum pressure during the respiratory cycle in the alveolus. At the beginning of a breath, alveolar pressure is at its lowest. During inspiration, as air fills the alveolus, pressure within the alveolus rises, reaching a maximum level

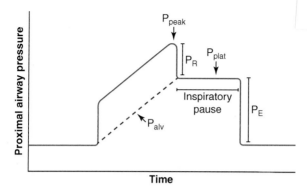

FIGURE 4.2 Pressure waveform with an inspiratory pause maneuver. This pressure waveform is from a volume-controlled ventilation mode with a constant flow waveform. Peak airway pressure is the maximum proximal airway pressure during the respiratory cycle. When an inspiratory pause maneuver is performed, inspiratory flow ceases and exhalation is temporarily prevented. Because flow has ceased, the resistive component of proximal airway pressure (P_R) becomes zero, making the measured proximal airway pressure equal to the elastic component (P_E). P_E at the end of inspiration is equal to plateau pressure. Note that alveolar pressure is at its lowest value at the beginning of inspiration and rises to its maximum level by the end of inspiration, which is equal to plateau pressure.

P_{air} proximal airway pressure; P_{alv} alveolar pressure; P_E elastic component of proximal airway pressure; P_{peak} peak airway pressure; P_{plat} plateau pressure; P_R resistive component of proximal airway pressure

once the entire tidal volume is delivered. That maximum level for alveolar pressure is equal to plateau pressure (Fig. 4.2).

Key Concept #3
Plateau pressure:

- Measure of maximum alveolar pressure during respiratory cycle
- Measured by **inspiratory pause maneuver**
- Higher with increased tidal volume and decreased respiratory system compliance

Diagnostic Algorithm

Peak and plateau pressures, as measured during VCV, can provide information about a patient's respiratory mechanics (Fig. 4.3). Elevated peak pressure is the result of elevated pressure from the resistive component, an elevated pressure from the elastic component, or both. To determine the etiology of elevated peak pressure, an inspiratory pause should be performed to measure plateau pressure. If plateau pressure is normal, the elevated peak pressure is due to increased airway resistance (Fig. 4.3b). Common causes of increased airway resistance include biting of the endotracheal tube, secretions in the airway, and bronchoconstriction. If plateau pressure is elevated, the elevated peak pressure is due to decreased respiratory system compliance or to increased lung volume (Fig. 4.3c). Common causes of decreased respiratory system compliance include pulmonary edema, pulmonary fibrosis, ascites, obesity, and pregnancy. Pneumothorax and atelectasis increase plateau pressure because the set tidal volume from VCV has less lung available to enter. Gas trapping, as explained in Chap. 6, also increases plateau pressure by increasing the end-expiratory lung volume and pressure—the addition of a set tidal volume to an elevated end-expiratory lung volume and pressure will result in elevated plateau pressure.

---➤

Figure 4.3 Pressure waveforms with inspiratory pause maneuver. (**a**) Normal peak and plateau pressure. (**b**) Elevated peak pressure but normal plateau pressure. The increased peak pressure is due to elevation in the resistive component of proximal airway pressure (P_R). (**c**) Elevated peak pressure and elevated plateau pressure. The increased peak pressure is due to an elevation in the elastic component of proximal airway pressure (P_E).

P_E elastic component of proximal airway pressure; P_{peak} peak airway pressure; P_{plat} plateau pressure; P_R resistive component of proximal airway pressure

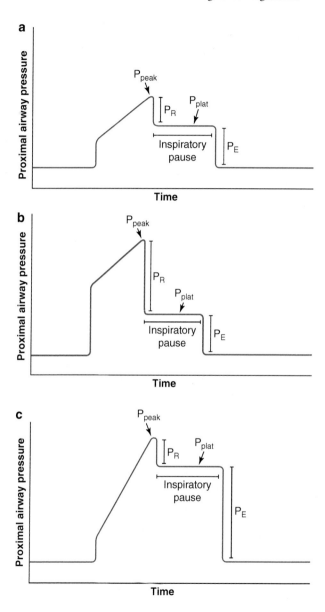

Key Concept #4
Causes of increased airway resistance:

- Biting of endotracheal tube
- Airway secretions
- Bronchoconstriction

Key Concept #5
Causes of decreased respiratory system compliance:

- Pulmonary edema
- Pulmonary fibrosis
- Pneumothorax
- Atelectasis
- Gas trapping
- Ascites
- Obesity
- Pregnancy

Decreased peak pressure during VCV can be noted in the setting of patient inspiratory efforts or an endotracheal tube cuff leak. Because flow in VCV is set, patient inspiratory efforts will not alter flow but will reduce proximal airway pressure. Apposition of the endotracheal tube cuff to the trachea seals the upper airway, allowing for pressurization of the respiratory system during inspiration. If the cuff does not form an adequate seal, air can leak outward, reducing peak airway pressure. Cuff leaks can occur because of cuff under-inflation, cephalad migration of the endotracheal tube, inadvertent intratracheal placement of a gastric tube, or a defective endotracheal tube cuff (Fig. 4.4).

Key Concept #6
Causes of decreased peak airway pressure:

- Patient inspiratory efforts
- Endotracheal tube cuff leak

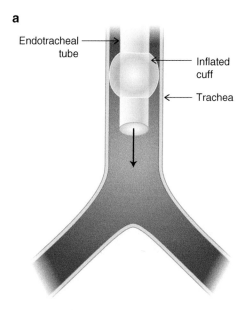

Figure 4.4 Endotracheal tube in the trachea. (**a**) The inflated cuff seals the upper airway and allows for pressurization of the respiratory system during inspiration. (**b**) An underinflated cuff results in air leak around the cuff and out of the upper airway, leading to lower proximal airway pressure with volume-controlled ventilation.

b

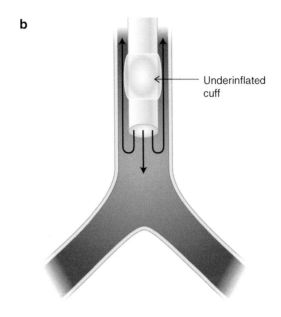

Underinflated cuff

FIGURE 4.4 (continued)

Suggested Readings

1. Cairo J. Pilbeam's mechanical ventilation: physiological and clinical applications. 5th ed. St. Louis: Mosby; 2012.
2. Hess D. Respiratory mechanics in mechanically ventilated patients. Respir Care. 2014;59:1773–94.
3. MacIntyre N, Branson R. Mechanical ventilation. 2nd ed. Philadelphia: Saunders; 2009.
4. Marino P. Marino's the ICU book. 3rd ed. Philadelphia: Lippincott Williams & Wilkins; 2007.
5. Tobin M. Principles and practice of mechanical ventilation. 3rd ed. Beijing: McGraw-Hill; 2013.

Chapter 5
Acute Respiratory Distress Syndrome

Acute respiratory distress syndrome (ARDS) is a syndrome characterized by increased permeability pulmonary edema, lung inflammation, hypoxemia, and decreased lung compliance. Clinical criteria include bilateral opacities on chest imaging, hypoxemia with a PaO_2/F_IO_2 ratio < 300 mm Hg with **positive end-expiratory pressure (PEEP)** ≥ 5 cm H_2O, and the respiratory failure cannot fully be explained by cardiac failure or fluid overload. Causes of ARDS can be categorized into those resulting from direct injury to the lungs (e.g., pneumonia, aspiration, toxic inhalation, near-drowning) and those from indirect injury to the lungs (e.g., sepsis, trauma, pancreatitis, blood transfusions). Lung inflammation in ARDS causes alveolar injury, leaky pulmonary capillaries, exudation of proteinaceous fluid into alveoli, and alveolar collapse. Patients with ARDS often require mechanical ventilation because of the increased work of breathing from decreased lung compliance and impaired gas exchange.

© Springer International Publishing AG,
part of Springer Nature 2018
H. Poor, *Basics of Mechanical Ventilation*,
https://doi.org/10.1007/978-3-319-89981-7_5

Key Concept #1
ARDS criteria:

- Acute
- Bilateral opacities
- PaO_2/F_IO_2 ratio < 300 mm Hg with PEEP $\geq$ 5 cm H_2O
- Infiltrates not completely explained by cardiac failure or fluid overload

Besides treating the underlying etiology, the treatment of ARDS is predominantly supportive. The goal is to allow time for the injured lung parenchyma to properly heal while avoiding damage to the uninjured lung. While mechanical ventilation is often critically necessary to sustain ventilation and gas exchange in patients with ARDS, the use of positive pressure ventilation can paradoxically worsen lung inflammation and damage. Three types of ventilator-induced lung injury have been described: **volutrauma**, **barotrauma**, and **atelectrauma**. Ventilator strategies employed in ARDS are primarily used to minimize these types of lung injury.

Volutrauma

Higher tidal volumes result in increased stretch of the lung parenchyma. This increased stretch, in the setting of already damaged lung parenchyma, results in further inflammation and lung injury. In a large multicenter, randomized controlled trial, the use of a low tidal volume strategy of 6 mL per kg of ideal body weight in patients with ARDS compared with larger tidal volumes resulted in a reduction in mortality. Ideal body weight, not actual body weight, is used to calculate the tidal volume because lung size is better correlated with height than actual weight—adult lungs do not grow with weight gain.

Key Concept #2
Tidal volume should be ≤ 6 mL per kg of ideal body
weight to prevent **volutrauma** in ARDS

Both volume and pressure modes of ventilation can be
used for low tidal volume ventilation. As discussed in Chap.
3, with volume-controlled ventilation (VCV), flow (target)
and volume (cycle) are set; therefore, changes in the patient's
lung compliance, airway resistance, and patient effort will
affect proximal airway pressure and not the delivered tidal
volume. For example, the development of strong inspiratory
efforts by the patient during VCV will not alter tidal volume
but will instead decrease proximal airway pressure.

With pressure-controlled ventilation (PCV), the target variable is proximal airway pressure, and the cycle variable is time.
Tidal volume, not directly set in this mode of ventilation, is
determined by proximal airway pressure, inspiratory time, and
characteristics of the respiratory system (lung compliance, airway resistance, and patient effort). Changes in the respiratory
system will not alter proximal airway pressure but will instead
affect flow and consequently tidal volume. For example, the
development of strong inspiratory efforts by the patient during
PCV will not alter proximal airway pressure and will instead
lead to increased inspiratory flow and consequently increased
tidal volume. In this case, tidal volume can be reduced by
decreasing proximal airway pressure. If PCV is used for
patients with ARDS, it is crucial that the resultant tidal volume
be closely monitored to ensure that lung overinflation does not
occur in the setting of changes in the respiratory system.

Barotrauma

Endotracheal tubes and the muscular cartilaginous airways
can withstand high airway pressure; however, excessive airway pressure in the alveoli can lead to complications such as

pneumothorax, pneumomediastinum, and subcutaneous emphysema. As explained in Chap. 4, plateau pressure can be viewed as the maximum pressure during the respiratory cycle in the alveolus; preventing high plateau pressure is important in the management of ARDS. To achieve lower plateau pressure with VCV, tidal volume must be reduced. For patients with very low lung compliance, tidal volume below 6 mL per kg may be necessary to achieve an acceptable plateau pressure. The goal plateau pressure is usually below 30 cm H_2O.

With PCV, flow is administered to quickly achieve and maintain the set proximal airway pressure. As air flows into the patient, alveolar pressure rises, and less flow is needed to achieve the set proximal airway pressure. If the inspiratory time (cycle) is long enough for flow to cease altogether, alveolar pressure will equal proximal airway pressure. Thus, setting lower proximal airway pressure will ensure lower alveolar pressure and help prevent barotrauma.

Atelectrauma

Alveolar collapse is a hallmark of ARDS. The repetitive opening and closing of collapsed alveoli with mechanical ventilation is detrimental, as high sheer stresses are generated at the interface of collapsed and aerated tissue when a collapsed alveolus is reopened. The lung injury that is perpetuated by this repetitive opening and closing of alveoli is known as atelectrauma. Surfactant is a substance that reduces alveolar wall surface tension, preventing alveolar collapse. Because of alveolar epithelial damage and inflammation, there are both a decrease in surfactant production and also a decrease in surfactant function, resulting in alveolar collapse and atelectasis.

The use of increased PEEP can minimize atelectrauma. As discussed in Chap. 1, PEEP is setting proximal airway pressure to be positive during the expiratory phase. **Opening pressure**, which is the minimum pressure required to open a closed alveolus, is higher than **closing pressure**, which is the

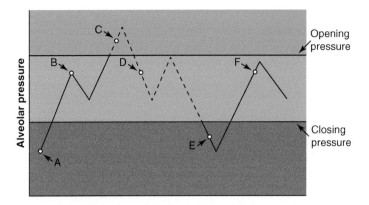

FIGURE 5.1 Schematic of an alveolus with varying alveolar pressure. The solid line represents the alveolus in a closed state, and the dotted line represents the alveolus in an open state. Note that alveolar pressure at Point B, Point D, and Point F is the same, but the alveolus is closed at Point B and Point F and open at Point D. Setting PEEP above closing pressure will prevent open alveoli from closing. *PEEP* positive end-expiratory pressure

minimum pressure required within an open alveolus to keep it open. That is, more force is needed to separate alveolar walls that have become stuck to each other than is needed to prevent alveolar walls from closing in the first place. Figure 5.1 demonstrates the relationship between alveolar pressure and the state of the alveolus. An alveolus with alveolar pressure below closing pressure will be closed (Point A). If alveolar pressure is increased to above closing pressure, but still below opening pressure, the alveolus remains closed as it has not risen above opening pressure (Point B). The alveolus will open only once alveolar pressure has increased to above opening pressure (Point C). After the alveolus has opened, if alveolar pressure is reduced to below opening pressure, yet still above closing pressure, the alveolus remains open (Point D). If alveolar pressure is then reduced below closing pressure, the alveolus will close (Point E). If alveolar pressure is again increased above closing pressure, but still below opening pressure, the alveolus remains closed (Point F). Note that alveolar pressure at Point B, Point D, and Point F is the same, yet the alveolus is closed at Point B and Point F and open at Point D. Theoretically, setting PEEP above closing pressure will prevent open alveoli from closing and will reduce atelectrauma.

Not only would setting PEEP above closing pressure of

Key Concept #3
- **Atelectrauma:** lung injury from repetitive opening and closing of alveoli
- PEEP can minimize atelectrauma by preventing closure of open alveoli

the alveoli prevent atelectrauma, it may maintain alveoli in an open state that would otherwise remain collapsed during the entire respiratory cycle. Because these open alveoli can now receive part of the delivered tidal volume, lung compliance may improve. These open alveoli can now participate in gas exchange, improving hypoxemia. It is important to note that PEEP does not actually "open" closed alveoli, but if set above closing pressure, it can prevent open alveoli from closing. In order to actually open a closed alveolus, alveolar pressure must exceed opening pressure. Recruitment maneuvers, which are transient increases in alveolar pressure that are intended to exceed opening pressure, can be utilized to open collapsed alveoli. While recruitment maneuvers have been shown to improve oxygenation in patients with ARDS, they have not been shown to improve clinically important outcomes like mortality or hospital length of stay.

PEEP can also have detrimental effects, particularly if it is not effective in preventing alveolar collapse and atelectasis. To illustrate this phenomenon, imagine that the administration of PEEP for a given patient does not lead to more alveoli remaining open. In this case, PEEP raises end-expiratory pressure of the open alveoli and thus increases their end-expiratory volume. This increased end-expiratory volume places these alveoli on a less compliant portion of the pressure-volume curve because lungs are less compliant at higher volumes (Fig. 1.4). Given that the administration of PEEP did not result in more alveoli remaining open for this patient, the entire tidal volume will be delivered to the same set of open alveoli. Since these alveoli are starting at an elevated *end-expiratory* volume and pressure, they will end at an elevated *end-inspiratory* volume and pressure. This alveolar overdistension can cause barotrauma and lung injury. Additionally, overdistended alveoli may compress their associated capillaries, shunting blood away from open, well-ventilated alveoli to collapsed, poorly ventilated alveoli. This shunted blood does not participate in gas exchange and, in fact, worsens hypoxemia (Fig. 5.2).

> **Key Concept #4**
> PEEP may paradoxically worsen gas exchange and decrease lung compliance by causing alveolar overdistension

Permissive Hypercapnia

The total amount of air that is inhaled and exhaled per minute, minute ventilation $\left(\dot{V}_E \right)$, is equal to tidal volume (V_T) multiplied by respiratory rate (RR):

$$\dot{V}_E = V_T \times RR$$

Minute ventilation is comprised of air that participates in gas exchange, known as alveolar ventilation $\left(\dot{V}_A \right)$, and air that does not participate in gas exchange, known as dead-space ventilation $\left(\dot{V}_D \right)$:

$$\dot{V}_E = \dot{V}_A + \dot{V}_D$$

Because alveolar ventilation is the amount of air that participates in gas exchange per unit time, the arterial partial pressure of carbon dioxide ($PaCO_2$) is inversely proportional to alveolar ventilation:

$$PaCO_2 \; \alpha \; \frac{1}{\dot{V}_A}$$

Therefore, with increased alveolar ventilation, $PaCO_2$ is low, while with decreased alveolar ventilation, $PaCO_2$ is high.

Employing a low tidal volume strategy in ARDS will result in decreased minute ventilation if the respiratory rate is not increased. A decreased minute ventilation will lead to decreased alveolar ventilation, which will result in elevated $PaCO_2$ and respiratory acidosis. When low tidal volume ventilation is utilized, the respiratory rate should be increased to compensate for the reduction in alveolar ventilation. However, because a certain amount of time is necessary for inspiration, there is a limit to how high the respiratory rate

Figure 5.2 Two alveolus model of the potential effect of increased PEEP on alveolar compliance and alveolar perfusion. (**a**) Without increased PEEP, the alveolus on the right remains open, while the alveolus on the left remains closed. Assuming the closed alveolus has high opening pressure, the entire tidal volume with inspiration will enter only the open alveolus, leading to high end-inspiratory (plateau) pressure. The closed alveolus does not participate in gas exchange with the capillary. (**b**) If increased PEEP maintains the collapsed alveolus open, both alveoli remain open at the end of expiration. The entire tidal volume with inspiration will be distributed between the two alveoli, improving overall lung compliance and possibly reducing end-inspiratory (plateau) pressure. Both alveoli participate in gas exchange with the capillaries. (**c**) If increased PEEP does not result in keeping the closed alveolus open, it may cause overdistension of the already open alveolus with resultant compression of its associated capillary, leading to shunting of blood to the collapsed, poorly ventilated alveolus.
PEEP positive end-expiratory pressure

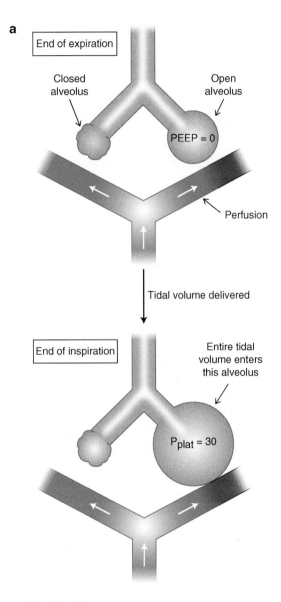

FIGURE 5.2 (continued)

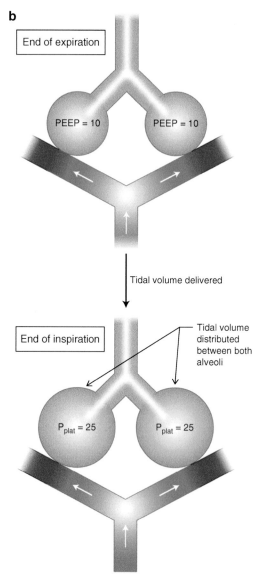

FIGURE 5.2 (continued)

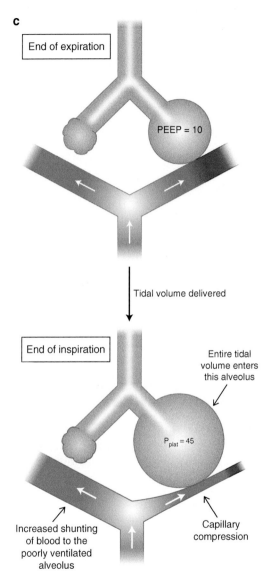

FIGURE 5.2 (continued)

can be set. **Permissive hypercapnia** refers to hypercapnia despite the maximum possible respiratory rate in the setting of low tidal volume ventilation. This increased $PaCO_2$, a result of low alveolar ventilation because of low tidal volume, is "permitted" because of the known benefits of maintaining low tidal volume in the setting of ARDS. Because low tidal volume ventilation may lead to patient discomfort and resultant patient-ventilator dyssynchrony, substantial sedation and even paralysis may be necessary.

Key Concept #5
Permissive hypercapnia: allowing elevated $PaCO_2$ because of benefit from low tidal volume ventilation

---

Suggested Readings

1. Brower R, Matthay M, Morris A, et al. Ventilation with lower tidal volumes as compared with traditional tidal volumes for acute lung injury and the acute respiratory distress syndrome. N Engl J Med. 2000;342:1301–8.
2. Cairo J. Pilbeam's mechanical ventilation: physiological and clinical applications. 5th ed. St. Louis: Mosby; 2012.
3. MacIntyre N, Branson R. Mechanical ventilation. 2nd ed. Philadelphia: Saunders; 2009.
4. Broaddus V, Ernst J. Murray and Nadel's textbook of respiratory medicine. 5th ed. Philadelphia: Saunders; 2010.
5. Schmidt G. Managing acute lung injury. Clin Chest Med. 2016;37:647–58.
6. Tobin M. Principles and practice of mechanical ventilation. 3rd ed. Beijing: McGraw-Hill; 2013.
7. West J. Pulmonary pathophysiology: the essentials. 8th ed. Beijing: Lippincott Williams & Wilkins; 2013.

Chapter 6
Obstructive Lung Diseases

Mechanical ventilation is often used in the setting of acute exacerbations of obstructive lung diseases like asthma and chronic obstructive pulmonary disease (COPD). These disorders are characterized by increased airway resistance secondary to bronchospasm and airway inflammation, collapse, and remodeling, often leading to inefficient exhalation and expiratory flow limitation. Patients with obstructive lung disease and inefficient exhalation require a longer expiratory time to achieve full exhalation.

Breath Stacking and Auto-PEEP

Mechanical ventilation in patients with inefficient exhalation can be challenging as patients may not achieve full exhalation prior to the triggering of another breath, a phenomenon known as **breath stacking**. In the setting of breath stacking, because full exhalation has not occurred, additional air remains within the alveoli at the end of expiration, a phenomenon known as **gas trapping**. Increased air within the alveoli at the end of expiration increases end-expiratory pressure, a phenomenon known as **auto-PEEP** (Fig. 6.1).

© Springer International Publishing AG,   61
part of Springer Nature 2018
H. Poor, *Basics of Mechanical Ventilation*,
https://doi.org/10.1007/978-3-319-89981-7_6

> **Key Concept #1**
> - **Breath stacking:** triggering another breath before complete exhalation
> - **Gas trapping:** retention of extra air in alveoli at end of expiration because of incomplete exhalation
> - **Auto-PEEP:** increase in alveolar end-expiratory pressure due to gas trapping

FIGURE 6.1 Effect of significantly increased airway resistance on exhalation. (**a**) Example of expiration in the setting of normal airway resistance. At the end of inspiration, alveolar pressure is 20 cm H_2O. At the beginning of expiration, proximal airway pressure is reduced to 5 cm H_2O (PEEP set on the ventilator). Because a pressure gradient exists between the alveolus and the proximal airway, air flows from the alveolus to the ventilator. In the setting of normal airway resistance, expiratory flow is fast enough for the alveolus to empty out a sufficient amount of air to reduce alveolar pressure to the level of proximal airway pressure. Note that if further time were allotted for expiration, no additional air would exit the alveolus, as no pressure gradient exists at the end of expiration between alveolar pressure and proximal airway pressure. (**b**) Example of expiration in the setting of significantly increased airway resistance. At the end of inspiration, alveolar pressure is 40 cm H_2O. At the beginning of expiration, proximal airway pressure is reduced to 5 cm H_2O (PEEP set on the ventilator). Because a pressure gradient exists between the alveolus and the proximal airway, air flows from the alveolus to the ventilator. In the setting of increased airway resistance, expiratory flow is slow—the alveolus is not able to empty out enough air to reduce alveolar pressure to the level of proximal airway pressure within the time allowed for expiration. The resultant increased alveolar pressure at the end of expiration is known as "auto-PEEP." Note that if further time were allotted for expiration, additional air would leave the alveolus because alveolar pressure at the end of expiration is still higher than proximal airway pressure.

P_{air} proximal airway pressure; P_{alv} alveolar pressure; *PEEP* positive end-expiratory pressure

Breath stacking and gas trapping increase end-expiratory alveolar pressure and volume; therefore, inspiration begins at already higher than normal lung volume and pressure. The administration of a set tidal volume (as occurs with volume-controlled ventilation) to lungs that have elevated end-expiratory volume and pressure results in elevated end-inspiratory lung volume and pressure. If breath stacking and gas trapping are severe enough, barotrauma may result from the increased pressure in the airways and the alveoli. Additionally, the increased intrathoracic pressure may compress cardiac structures, decreasing venous return to the heart and ultimately leading to hemodynamic compromise and even obstructive shock.

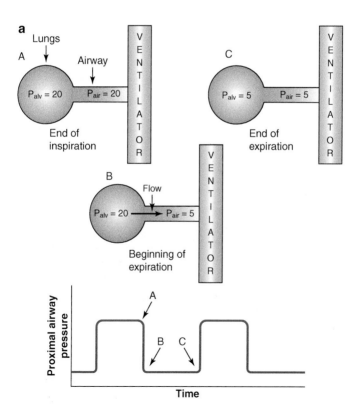

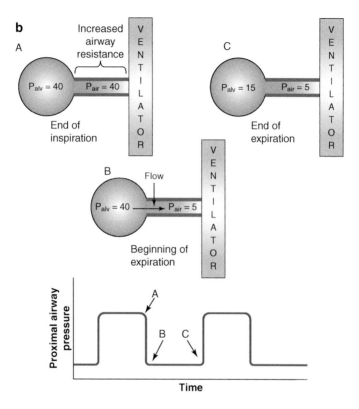

FIGURE 6.1 (continued)

As discussed in Chap. 4, elevated plateau pressure can suggest the presence of elevated end-inspiratory lung volume and hyperinflation in the setting of obstructive lung disease. In pressure-targeted modes (pressure-controlled ventilation and pressure support ventilation), where flow is administered to quickly achieve and maintain a set inspiratory pressure, the presence of elevated end-expiratory volume and pressure results in decreased tidal volume—less flow and volume will be needed to achieve the set inspiratory pressure, which can ultimately result in hypoventilation.

Key Concept #2
Elevated plateau pressure can signify hyperinflation in the setting of obstructive lung disease

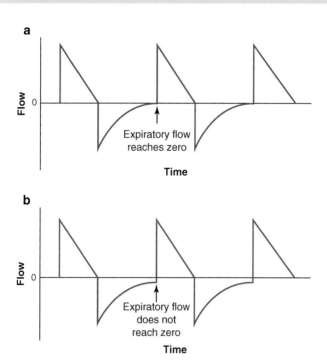

FIG. 6.2 Flow waveform patterns. (**a**) Normal expiratory flow pattern. Note that expiratory flow reaches zero prior to the initiation of the subsequent breath. (**b**) Expiratory flow pattern demonstrating breath stacking. Note that expiratory flow does not reach zero prior to the initiation of the subsequent breath. The presence of expiratory flow at the end of expiration implies that alveolar pressure is higher than proximal airway pressure at that time point.

Evaluation of the expiratory flow curve on the ventilator can aid in the identification of breath stacking (Fig. 6.2). Under normal conditions, the expiratory portion of the flow curve should return to zero before the end of expiration, indicating that expiratory flow has ceased. If a breath is triggered and administered before expiratory flow has reached zero, breath stacking is present.

Breath stacking can also be identified by listening to lung sounds. In order for wheezing to occur, flow must be present. Expiratory wheezing up until the very last moment prior to the subsequent breath being triggered indicates that expiratory flow has not reached zero at end-expiration and that breath stacking is present.

Key Concept #3
Identifying breath stacking:

- Expiratory flow does not reach zero at end of expiration
- Wheezing persists right up to initiation of subsequent breath

---

The magnitude of auto-PEEP can also be assessed by employing an **expiratory pause maneuver** on the ventilator (Fig. 6.3). With this maneuver, the expiratory valve is closed at the end of expiration, not allowing any additional air to leave the respiratory system. If, at the end of expiration, alveolar pressure is still higher than proximal airway pressure (PEEP applied at the ventilator), air will continue to flow from the alveoli to the ventilator, raising proximal airway pressure. The amount that proximal airway pressure rises above PEEP applied at the ventilator is referred to as auto-PEEP or **intrinsic PEEP**. Of note, PEEP applied at the ventilator is often referred to as **applied PEEP** or **extrinsic PEEP**. Total PEEP is equal to the sum of intrinsic PEEP and extrinsic PEEP. It is important that the expiratory pause maneuver be performed on a patient who is not making respiratory efforts—patient inspiratory and expiratory efforts will change the measured pressure and will not properly reflect the presence or degree of auto-PEEP.

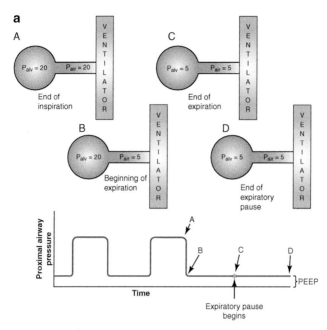

FIGURE 6.3 Expiratory pause maneuver demonstrating auto-PEEP. (a) Example of expiratory pause maneuver in the setting of normal airway resistance. At the end of expiration, the expiratory valve closes, not allowing any air to leave the respiratory system. Because alveolar pressure equals proximal airway pressure at the end of expiration, there is no additional flow from the alveolus to the ventilator; therefore, proximal airway pressure remains unchanged at the end of the expiratory pause maneuver, and there is no intrinsic PEEP. Total PEEP is thus equal to extrinsic PEEP. (b) Example of expiratory pause maneuver in the setting of significantly increased airway resistance. At the end of expiration, the expiratory valve closes, not allowing any air to leave the respiratory system. Because alveolar pressure is still higher than proximal airway pressure at the end of expiration, there is additional flow from the alveolus to the ventilator, which continues to increase proximal airway pressure. The additional increase in proximal airway pressure at the end of expiration is known as "intrinsic PEEP" or "auto-PEEP." In this case, intrinsic PEEP is 7 cm H_2O, extrinsic PEEP is 5 cm H_2O, and total PEEP is 12 cm H_2O. P_{air} proximal airway pressure; P_{alv} alveolar pressure; *PEEP* positive end-expiratory pressure; $PEEP_e$ extrinsic positive end-expiratory pressure; $PEEP_i$ intrinsic positive end-expiratory pressure

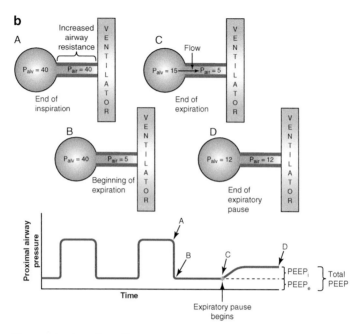

FIGURE 6.3 (continued)

> **Key Concept #4**
> Magnitude of auto-PEEP can be assessed with the **expiratory pause maneuver**

Ventilator Management Strategies

The central principle in managing patients on the ventilator with obstructive lung disease and expiratory flow limitation is to increase the time allowed for exhalation and to decrease tidal volume so that less air needs to be exhaled. By increasing the expiratory time, there is a greater chance that expiratory flow will reach zero prior to the subsequent breath,

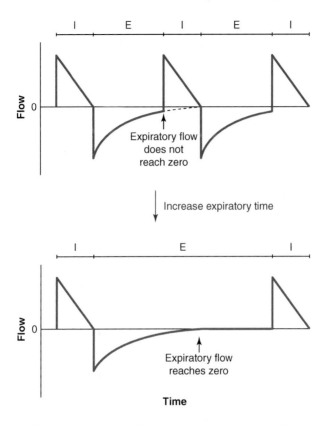

FIGURE 6.4 Flow waveforms demonstrating that gas trapping can be diminished by increasing time for expiration. Note that expiratory flow does not reach zero prior to the subsequent breath in the top diagram but in the lower diagram, with increased time for expiration, expiratory flow does reach zero.

decreasing the degree of gas trapping, auto-PEEP, and hyperinflation (Fig. 6.4).

From the perspective of the ventilator, expiration is defined as the time during the respiratory cycle that is not inspiration. Specifically, it is the time between when one breath cycles off and the next breath is triggered. The relative time a patient spends in inspiration versus expiration is known as the **inspiration:expiration ratio (I:E ratio)**. Patients with obstructive lung disease and expiratory flow limitation undergoing mechanical ventilation benefit from low I:E ratios in order to maximize expiratory time. A patient can be in only one of two phases of the respiratory cycle: inspiratory or expiratory. By decreasing the overall time spent in inspiration, expiratory time increases and the I:E ratio decreases. Time spent in inspiration can be decreased by either decreasing the inspiratory time per breath (i.e., reducing the time it takes to deliver each breath) or by reducing the number of inspirations per unit time (i.e., reducing the respiratory rate) (Fig. 6.5).

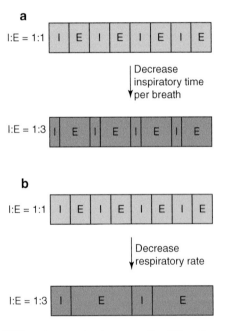

Figure 6.5 Different ways to decrease the I:E ratio and increase expiratory time. (**a**) Total inspiratory time and I:E ratio decreased by reducing inspiratory time per breath. (**b**) Total inspiratory time and I:E ratio decreased by reducing respiratory rate. E expiration; I inspiration

While low respiratory rate and tidal volume are optimal for managing patients with expiratory flow limitation, utilizing this strategy will often result in hypoventilation and hypercapnia. This permissive hypercapnia is allowed because of the benefits of preventing breath stacking, auto-PEEP, and hyperinflation. Permissive hypercapnia is also utilized in the management of ARDS with low tidal volume ventilation (Chap. 5).

Assist-Control

For modes of ventilation that use an assist-control trigger (volume-controlled ventilation or pressure-controlled ventilation), decreasing the set respiratory rate will reduce total inspiratory time and therefore increase expiratory time. For example, if a patient's respiratory rate is 20 breaths per minute with an inspiratory time of 1 second per breath, the patient is spending a total of 20 seconds per minute in the inspiratory phase. Therefore, the patient is spending 40 seconds per minute in the expiratory phase, which equates to 2 seconds per expiratory cycle. Decreasing the respiratory rate to 10 breaths per minute would result in the patient spending a total of 10 seconds per minute in the inspiratory phase and thus a total of 50 seconds per minute in the expiratory phase, which equates to 5 seconds per expiratory cycle. The respiratory rate can be reduced using the ventilator only if the breaths are ventilator-triggered breaths. Reducing the respiratory rate for a patient who has exclusively patient-triggered breaths will not affect the respiratory rate. In these scenarios, sedation, and even paralysis, may be necessary to reduce the respiratory rate.

Volume-Controlled Ventilation

As previously discussed, in volume-controlled ventilation, the target is flow, and the cycle is volume. Increasing flow reduces the time required to deliver the set tidal volume, which reduces inspiratory time for each breath. Decreasing inspirary time for each breath will then increase expiratory time. Note that, based on the equation from Chap. 4, increasing flow will also increase proximal airway pressure:

$$P_{air} = Q \times R + \frac{V}{C}$$

C = compliance
Q = flow
P_{air} = proximal airway pressure
R = airway resistance
V = volume

However, most of this pressure is dissipated in the endotracheal tube and central airways, which can withstand this increased pressure. Alveolar pressure will not be affected if tidal volume remains the same.

Decreasing tidal volume will also increase expiratory time. By decreasing volume, less time is needed for inspiration at a given flow, resulting in an increase in expiratory time. Additionally, with decreased tidal volume, less time is needed to fully expire the total administered tidal volume.

> **Key Concept #5**
> Ventilator strategies to increase expiratory time in VCV:
>
> - Decrease respiratory rate
> - Decrease tidal volume
> - Increase flow rate

Pressure-Controlled Ventilation

In pressure-controlled ventilation, the target is proximal airway pressure, and the cycle is time. Inspiratory time can be directly reduced, leading to an increase in expiratory time. Tidal volume can be reduced by decreasing proximal airway pressure. With decreased tidal volume, less time is needed to fully expire the total administered tidal volume.

Pressure Support Ventilation

In pressure support ventilation, the target is proximal airway pressure, and the cycle is flow. Similar to pressure-controlled ventilation, proximal airway pressure can be reduced, which decreases tidal volume. Inspiratory time can be decreased by increasing the flow cycle threshold, which is the percentage of peak flow to which inspiratory flow must diminish in order for inspiration to be terminated. By increasing this threshold, flow does not have to reach as low a level, and inspiration will be terminated sooner, resulting in decreased inspiratory time. This decreased inspiratory time will also result in decreased tidal volume.

Suggested Readings

1. Bergin S, Rackley C. Managing respiratory failure in obstructive lung disease. Clin Chest Med. 2016;37:659–67.
2. Cairo J. Pilbeam's mechanical ventilation: physiological and clinical applications. 5th ed. St. Louis: Mosby; 2012.
3. MacIntyre N, Branson R. Mechanical ventilation. 2nd ed. Philadelphia: Saunders; 2009.
4. Broaddus V, Ernst J. Murray and Nadel's textbook of respiratory medicine. 5th ed. Philadelphia: Saunders; 2010.
5. Tobin M. Principles and practice of mechanical ventilation. 3rd ed. Beijing: McGraw-Hill; 2013.
6. West J. Pulmonary pathophysiology: the essentials. 8th ed. Beijing: Lippincott Williams & Wilkins; 2013.

Chapter 7
Patient-Ventilator Dyssynchrony

For patients receiving mechanical ventilation who are not using their respiratory muscles, all of the work of breathing is done by the ventilator. This scenario often occurs in the setting of deep sedation, paralysis, or significant neurologic dysfunction. However, many patients receiving mechanical ventilation are active participants in the respiratory process and use their respiratory muscles. The ventilator's role for these patients is to reduce the work of breathing. In order for this collaboration between the patient and the ventilator to occur successfully, a significant amount of synchrony is necessary for breath initiation (trigger), inspiratory flow determination (target), and breath termination (cycle). Dyssynchrony between the patient and the ventilator can result in significant patient discomfort and increased work of breathing. The types of dyssynchrony are characterized as those that occur during the trigger phase, the target phase, and the cycle phase.

Trigger-Related Dyssynchrony

As described in Chap. 2, patient-triggered breaths are initiated by patient respiratory efforts. These respiratory efforts alter pressure and flow in the respiratory circuit. With a pressure trigger, a breath is initiated when an inspiratory effort reduces proximal airway pressure by more than the set pressure thresh-

© Springer International Publishing AG,
part of Springer Nature 2018
H. Poor, *Basics of Mechanical Ventilation*,
https://doi.org/10.1007/978-3-319-89981-7_7

old on the ventilator (Fig. 2.2). For a flow trigger, a breath is initiated when an inspiratory effort draws a certain amount of the continuous ventilator flow away from the ventilator (Fig. 2.3). **Ineffective triggering**, sometimes called **missed triggering**, occurs when patient attempts to trigger the ventilator are unsuccessful. **Extra triggering** occurs when breaths are inappropriately triggered using the pressure or flow triggering mechanism in the absence of patient inspiratory effort.

Ineffective Triggering

A patient's inspiratory effort must achieve a set pressure or flow threshold in order to trigger a breath. Patients with severe respiratory weakness may be unable to reliably trigger breaths despite their respiratory efforts. This problem is exacerbated if the trigger threshold for either the pressure or the flow trigger is set too high, necessitating stronger respiratory efforts in order to trigger the ventilator. Furthermore, if using a flow trigger, the addition of extra flow to the circuit with continuous-flow nebulizer treatments can produce ineffective triggering. With a flow trigger, in order for the patient to successfully trigger the ventilator, the patient's respiratory effort must be strong enough to inspire all of the additional flow provided by the nebulizer, in addition to the threshold amount of continuous flow from the ventilator's inspiratory limb (Fig. 7.1).

Figure 7.1 Respiratory circuit demonstrating the flow trigger mechanism. (**a**) A continuous amount of gas flows from the inspiratory limb to the expiratory limb of the ventilator. (**b**) A patient's inspiratory effort will cause some of the gas flow to enter the patient instead of returning to the ventilator. If the reduction in flow returning to the ventilator is above the flow trigger threshold, the inspiratory effort would trigger the ventilator. (**c**) The use of continuous-flow nebulizer treatments adds additional flow into the inspiratory limb of the respiratory circuit. In order for the patient to successfully trigger the ventilator, the patient must inspire all of the flow delivered by the nebulizer, in addition to the threshold amount of continuous flow from the inspiratory limb of the ventilator that is destined for the expiratory limb.

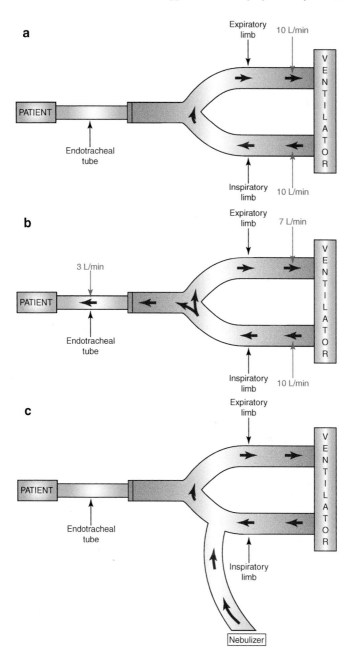

To avoid this problem, the trigger mechanism should be set to a pressure—not flow—trigger.

> **Key Concept #1**
> **Ineffective triggering:** patient inspiratory efforts do not trigger ventilator

Ineffective triggering can also develop in the setting of significant auto-PEEP (see Chap. 6). In patients with inefficient exhalation and expiratory flow limitation, full exhalation is not achieved prior to subsequent attempts to trigger a breath. Incomplete emptying causes alveolar pressure at the end of expiration to be higher than proximal airway pressure, a phenomenon known as intrinsic PEEP, or auto-PEEP. As discussed in Chap. 2, proximal airway pressure during expiration is equal to PEEP set on the ventilator. To successfully trigger the ventilator, the patient must reduce alveolar pressure below proximal airway pressure (PEEP set on the ventilator). This reduction in alveolar pressure below proximal airway pressure diverts flow away from the ventilator's expiratory limb (flow trigger) and reduces proximal airway pressure (pressure trigger). For a patient with auto-PEEP, a larger decrease in pleural pressure (which requires increased inspiratory strength) is needed to sufficiently reduce alveolar pressure below proximal airway pressure. Inability to sufficiently reduce alveolar pressure below proximal airway pressure leads to ineffective triggering. Additionally, patients with significant auto-PEEP often have hyperinflated lungs. Hyperinflated lungs flatten the diaphragm and put the muscles of respiration at a mechanical disadvantage, making them weaker and less able to properly trigger the ventilator (Fig. 7.2).

FIGURE 7.2 Auto-PEEP can lead to ineffective triggering. (**a**) Example of triggering in the setting of normal airway resistance and absence of auto-PEEP. Because airway resistance is normal, the alveolus is able to empty out enough air so that alveolar pressure is reduced to proximal airway pressure at the end of expiration. A patient inspiratory effort reduces pleural pressure, which in this example leads to a decrease in alveolar pressure by 5 cm H_2O and creates a pressure gradient between

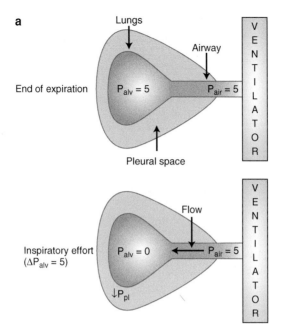

proximal airway pressure (PEEP set on the ventilator) and alveolar pressure. This pressure gradient causes air to flow from the ventilator into the patient, ultimately reducing proximal airway pressure. With a pressure trigger, a reduction in proximal airway pressure to a level below the threshold will trigger the ventilator. With a flow trigger, a flow rate into the patient that is above the threshold will trigger the ventilator. (**b**) Example of triggering in the setting of increased airway resistance. Because airway resistance is significantly elevated, the alveolus is not able to empty out enough air for alveolar pressure to be reduced to the level of proximal airway pressure in the allotted time, resulting in auto-PEEP. A patient inspiratory effort that reduces alveolar pressure by 5 cm H_2O will not reduce alveolar pressure to below the level of proximal airway pressure. Therefore, air does not flow from the ventilator into the patient, proximal airway pressure does not drop, and ultimately the patient inspiratory effort does not trigger a breath. A stronger inspiratory effort is necessary to trigger a breath in the setting of auto-PEEP. In this case, the inspiratory effort must reduce alveolar pressure by 15 cm H_2O in order to achieve the same gradient between proximal airway pressure and alveolar pressure that was achieved in example (**a**).

P_{air} proximal airway pressure; P_{alv} alveolar pressure; *PEEP* positive end-expiratory pressure; P_{pl} pleural pressure

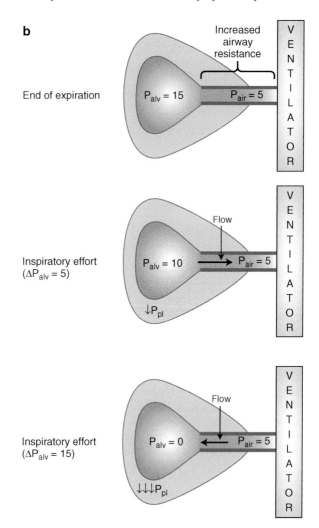

FIGURE 7.2 (continued)

Key Concept #2
Causes of ineffective triggering:

- Respiratory muscle weakness
- Trigger threshold set too high (decreased trigger sensitivity)
- Use of continuous-flow nebulizer with flow trigger
- Auto-PEEP

Management of ineffective triggering secondary to auto-PEEP is primarily to treat the underlying disorder that is causing increased airway resistance and expiratory flow limitation, usually with bronchodilators and other medications (e.g., corticosteroids). Ventilator-specific management should employ those strategies which minimize auto-PEEP as described in Chap. 6.

Increased airway resistance during expiration can be exacerbated by airway collapse during expiration, a phenomenon known as dynamic airway compression. As discussed in Chap. 1, expiration on the ventilator is generally passive. That is, no active contraction of respiratory muscles is required for expiration to occur. However, actively breathing patients may try to increase expiratory flow by using expiratory muscles to further increase pleural pressure and alveolar pressure. In patients with collapsible airways (e.g., COPD), this attempt to increase expiratory flow by increasing pleural pressure may be unsuccessful—the increased pleural pressure can compress the airways and result in airway collapse. The airway collapse is particularly pronounced near the end of expiration when lung volumes are lower and there is less tethering open of airways. This condition in which increasing expiratory effort does not increase the expiratory flow rate is known as **expiratory flow limitation** (Fig. 7.3).

Airway compression and collapse during expiration may result in a situation where there is no communication between the alveolus and the proximal airway. Because there is no communication between the alveolus and the proximal airway, increasing proximal airway pressure by increasing PEEP to a

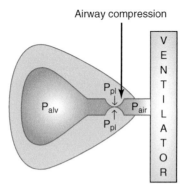

FIGURE 7.3 Airway collapse and expiratory flow limitation. In the setting of expiratory flow limitation, increasing alveolar pressure by increasing pleural pressure will not increase expiratory flow—the increase in alveolar pressure will be offset by the increased compressive force on the airway from elevated pleural pressure.
P_{air} proximal airway pressure; P_{alv} alveolar pressure; P_{pl} pleural pressure

critical pressure will not increase alveolar pressure. This scenario is analogous to a waterfall in a river—increasing the level of the river downstream to the waterfall will not increase the level of the river upstream as long as the level of the river downstream is lower than the level of the river upstream (Fig. 7.4).

In cases of ineffective triggering secondary to auto-PEEP, the addition of external PEEP to increase proximal airway pressure can reduce the work needed to trigger the ventilator if the increase in proximal airway pressure does not lead to increased alveolar pressure (i.e., the waterfall effect is present). By increasing proximal airway pressure without affecting alveolar pressure, the extent to which alveolar pressure needs to be lowered to trigger the ventilator is reduced (Fig. 7.5).

Key Concept #3
Ineffective triggering due to auto-PEEP can sometimes be reduced by adding external PEEP

If the additional external PEEP is transmitted to the alveolus (waterfall effect is not present), alveolar pressure is increased further. In this scenario, the work needed to trigger the ventilator is not reduced, and the increased alveolar pressure further worsens hyperinflation (Fig. 7.6).

Ineffective triggering can be detected by noting the activity of accessory inspiratory muscles (e.g., sternocleidomastoid

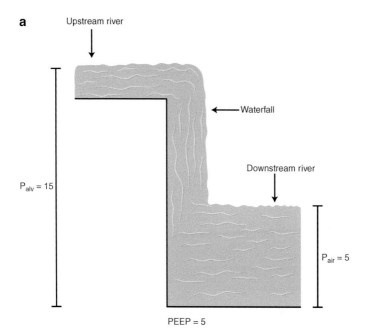

FIGURE 7.4 The "waterfall effect." Increasing the level of the downstream river will not affect the level of the upstream river as long as the level of the downstream river is lower than the level of the upstream river. The level of the downstream river is analogous to proximal airway pressure, and the level of the upstream river is analogous to alveolar pressure. In this example, if alveolar pressure is 15 cm H_2O and proximal airway pressure is 5 cm H_2O (a), increasing proximal airway pressure to 10 cm H_2O will not affect alveolar pressure (b). However, increasing proximal airway pressure to 20 cm H_2O will increase alveolar pressure to 20 cm H_2O (c).

P_{air} proximal airway pressure; P_{alv} alveolar pressure; PEEP positive end-expiratory pressure

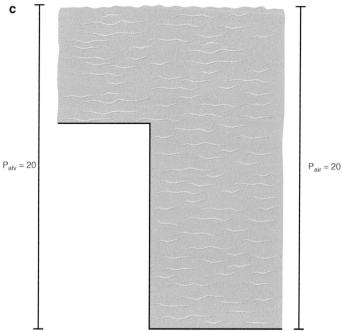

Fɪɢ. 4 (continued)

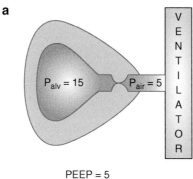

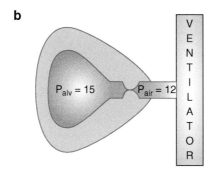

FIGURE 7.5 Increasing proximal airway pressure with external PEEP can decrease the inspiratory work needed to trigger the ventilator in the setting of auto-PEEP. (**a**) At the end of expiration, alveolar pressure is significantly higher than proximal airway pressure, indicating the presence of auto-PEEP. Assuming a gradient of 5 cm H_2O between proximal airway pressure and alveolar pressure is required to achieve the threshold pressure and/or flow changes to trigger the ventilator, the patient must reduce alveolar pressure down to 0 cm H_2O (reduction of 15 cm H_2O) in order to trigger the ventilator. (**b**) If external PEEP is increased to 12 cm H_2O from 5 cm H_2O, and the waterfall effect is present due to airway collapse, alveolar pressure will remain unchanged. The patient now only needs to reduce alveolar pressure to 7 cm H_2O (reduction of 8 cm H_2O) in order to trigger the ventilator, which requires less work.

P_{air} proximal airway pressure; P_{alv} alveolar pressure; PEEP positive end-expiratory pressure

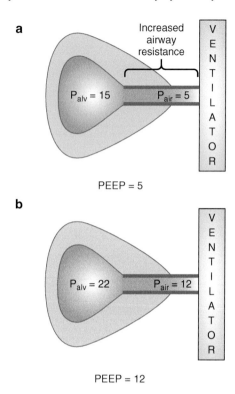

FIGURE 7.6 Increasing proximal airway pressure with external PEEP can be detrimental if dynamic airway compression is not present. (**a**) At the end of expiration, alveolar pressure is significantly higher than proximal airway pressure, indicating the presence of auto-PEEP. Assuming that a gradient of 5 cm H_2O between proximal airway pressure and alveolar pressure is needed to achieve the threshold pressure and/or flow changes to trigger the ventilator, the patient must reduce alveolar pressure down to 0 cm H_2O (reduction of 15 cm H_2O) in order to trigger the ventilator. (**b**) If external PEEP is increased to 12 cm H_2O from 5 cm H_2O, and the waterfall effect is not present, the additional pressure is transmitted to the alveolus, increasing alveolar pressure and worsening hyperinflation. The patient still needs to reduce alveolar pressure by 15 cm H_2O in order to trigger the ventilator.

P_{air} proximal airway pressure; P_{alv} alveolar pressure; PEEP positive end-expiratory pressure

and scalene muscles) without the triggering of the ventilator. More invasive techniques, such as diaphragmatic electromyography or measurement of pleural pressure using an esophageal probe, can be utilized as well.

> **Key Concept #4**
> Accessory inspiratory muscle activity that does not trigger the ventilator may indicate ineffective triggering

Extra Triggering

Extra triggering occurs when breaths are inappropriately triggered and are not reflective of the patient's intrinsic respiratory rate. This type of dyssynchrony can be further classified into **auto-triggering** or **double triggering**. Auto-triggering occurs in the setting of excessive condensation in the tubing that results in oscillations of water, small leaks in the circuit, or cardiac oscillations – all of these conditions result in changes in flow and pressure that can trigger the ventilator. Having a lower trigger threshold increases the chance that these oscillations will trigger a breath. Determining the best trigger threshold balances the risk of auto-triggering with the work the patient must do to trigger the breath. That is, the optimal trigger sensitivity is low enough that the patient triggers every breath with as little effort as possible but high enough to avoid auto-triggering.

> **Key Concept #5**
> - Trigger threshold too high → increased risk of ineffective triggering
> - Trigger threshold too low → increased risk of auto-triggering

Target-Related Dyssynchrony

The target variable determines how flow is delivered during inspiration. With flow-targeted modes like volume-controlled ventilation, flow is set and cannot be changed by patient respiratory efforts. A patient who makes increased inspiratory efforts due to a desire to increase flow will not affect the flow rate. Instead, those increased inspiratory efforts will result in a drop in proximal airway pressure, yielding a characteristic "scooping out" of the pressure curve, as discussed in Chap. 2 (Fig. 7.7).

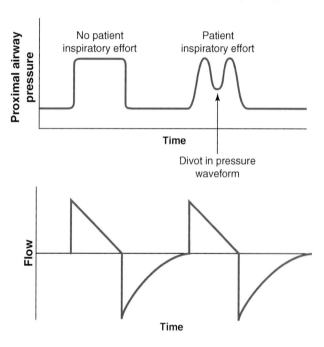

FIGURE 7.7 Flow and pressure waveforms of a flow-targeted mode demonstrating the response to a sustained patient inspiratory effort. A patient inspiratory effort, which decreases alveolar pressure, will not affect the flow waveform because the flow waveform is set in flow-targeted mode. Instead, there will be a decrease in proximal airway pressure during the inspiratory effort, as represented by a divot in the pressure waveform.

This mismatch between the patient's desired flow and machine-delivered flow can result in significant patient discomfort and even greater increases in inspiratory efforts. Flow dyssynchrony resulting from inadequate flow delivery can be addressed by either increasing the flow rate to match patient demands or by treating the underlying cause for increased flow demand (e.g., agitation or pain). Additionally, switching the mode to a pressure-targeted mode (pressure-controlled ventilation or pressure support ventilation) allows the patient to regulate flow. If utilizing this method, one must be cognizant of lung volume, as exuberant inspiratory efforts in pressure-targeted modes can result in very high volume, which may be deleterious.

Flow dyssynchrony can also occur in the setting of excessively high flow rate. Lung expansion at a rate faster than that desired by the patient's ventilatory control center can lead to activation of expiratory muscles and "fighting" or "bucking" the ventilator.

Cycle-Related Dyssynchrony

The cycle variable determines inspiratory phase duration. With normal spontaneous breathing, inspiration occurs because of a drop in pleural pressure due to contraction of inspiratory muscles. The duration of inspiratory muscle contraction leading to inspiration is known as the patient's **neural inspiratory time (neural T_I)**. Patient-ventilator dyssynchrony can occur when there is a mismatch between a patient's neural T_I and the cycle length, also known as the ventilator's T_I.

Premature cycling occurs when neural T_I is longer than the ventilator's T_I. This form of dyssynchrony can result in double triggering. In this situation, the patient continues to have sustained diaphragmatic contraction after the ventilator has cycled off inspiration. Since the ventilator is now in the expiratory (baseline) phase, the sustained diaphragmatic contraction and resultant drop in proximal airway pressure will immediately trigger another breath (Fig. 7.8).

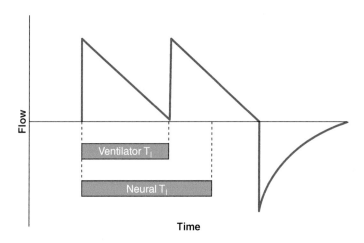

FIGURE 7.8 Flow waveform in volume-controlled ventilation demonstrating double triggering. In this case, the ventilator T_I is shorter than neural T_I. During neural T_I, the patient is contracting the inspiratory muscles, resulting in a reduction in pleural pressure and proximal airway pressure. Active patient inspiratory efforts during ventilator T_I do not trigger the ventilator and will instead decrease proximal airway pressure in flow-targeted modes and increase flow in pressure-targeted modes. However, active inspiratory efforts during expiration (after ventilator T_I has elapsed) can trigger the ventilator again. In this case, one patient inspiratory effort has triggered the ventilator twice. T_I inspiratory time

In volume-controlled ventilation, double triggering will result in two breaths being delivered without exhalation in between, which is essentially the delivery of one breath with double the tidal volume. This large tidal volume can be problematic. In acute respiratory distress syndrome, it can lead to volutrauma. In obstructive lung disease, it can worsen hyperinflation.

In pressure-controlled ventilation, double triggering will result in two breaths being delivered without exhalation in between. However, the tidal volume of the second breath will be much lower—less flow and volume will be necessary to achieve the set proximal airway pressure because there is already air in the lungs from the previous inspiration.

Double triggering can be addressed by increasing the ventilator's T_I. In volume-controlled ventilation, this can be achieved by decreasing the flow rate or by increasing tidal volume. Additionally, an end-inspiratory pause can be added—after the entire tidal volume has been delivered and flow has stopped, the expiratory valve is closed, and the lung remains at full inflation, during which another breath cannot be triggered. In pressure-controlled ventilation, inspiratory time can be increased. In pressure support ventilation, double triggering is not a common phenomenon because the cycle variable for PSV is flow (specifically, a diminishing to a set percentage of the peak flow). Lastly, if the ventilator settings are optimal and changes would increase the risk of harm, additional sedation, or even paralytics, can be administered.

Another form of double triggering is **entrainement**, also referred to as **reverse triggering**. Entrainment occurs when the administration of a control breath by the ventilator stimulates diaphragmatic contraction, resulting in the triggering of another breath immediately after the initial breath. A double triggering pattern which consists of a "control" breath immediately followed by an "assist" breath raises the suspicion of entrainment.

> **Key Concept #6**
> Suspect **entrainment** when double triggering pattern consists of **control** breath immediately followed by **assist** breath

Delayed cycling occurs when the ventilator's T_I is longer than the neural T_I. In this case, the ventilator is still in inspiration when the patient would like to be in expiration. In some cases, this can lead to significant patient discomfort, and patients may actively try to exhale during the time period when there is mismatch. In volume-controlled ventilation, this can be seen as notching of the pressure curve at the end of inspiration (Fig. 7.9).

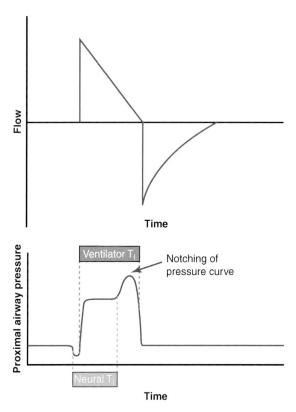

FIGURE 7.9 Flow and pressure waveforms in volume-controlled ventilation demonstrating delayed cycling. The beginning of neural T_I is marked by a negative deflection in the pressure waveform, indicating the contraction of inspiratory muscles, which decreases pleural pressure and proximal airway pressure. In this example, the ventilator terminates inspiration later than the patient does — ventilator T_I extends beyond the end of neural T_I. After neural T_I has elapsed, the patient attempts to actively exhale by contracting the expiratory muscles in order to further increase alveolar pressure; however, the beginning of this exhalation maneuver is occurring during the ventilator's inspiratory phase. Because the target in this mode of ventilation is flow, the flow waveform is not affected by the exhalation attempt, and instead proximal airway pressure rises, as noted by the notching at the end of the pressure curve.

T_I inspiratory time

Key Concept #7
- **Double triggering:** neural T_I > ventilator T_I
- **Delayed cycling:** neural T_I < ventilator T_I

Suggested Readings

1. Branson R, Blakeman T, Robinson B. Asynchrony and dyspnea. Respir Care. 2013;58:973–89.
2. Cairo J. Pilbeam's mechanical ventilation: physiological and clinical applications. 5th ed. St. Louis: Mosby; 2012.
3. Gentile M. Cycling of the mechanical ventilator breath. Respir Care. 2011;56:52–60.
4. Gilstrap D, MacIntyre N. Patient-ventilator interactions. Implications for clinical management. Am J Respir Crit Care Med. 2013;188:1058–68.
5. MacIntyre N, Branson R. Mechanical ventilation. 2nd ed. Philadelphia: Saunders; 2009.
6. Nilstestuen J, Hargett K. Using ventilator graphics to identify patient-ventilator asynchrony. Respir Care. 2005;52:202–34.
7. Tobin M, Lodato R. PEEP, auto-PEEP, and waterfalls. Chest. 1989;96:449–51.
8. Tobin M. Principles and practice of mechanical ventilation. 3rd ed. Beijing: McGraw-Hill; 2013.

Chapter 8
Indications for Mechanical Ventilation

The main indication for mechanical ventilation is respiratory failure, defined as the inability of the lungs to perform adequate gas exchange. Mechanical ventilators utilize positive pressure to support gas exchange and unload the muscles of respiration. This chapter will review some of the common causes of respiratory failure.

Increased Work of Breathing

As described in Chap. 4, the respiratory system can be broken down into two components: the resistive component and the elastic component. In spontaneously breathing patients, the muscles of respiration must make alveolar pressure substantially negative to draw air through the resistive component (airways) as well as inflate the elastic component (lungs and chest wall). If there is an increase in either airway resistance or lung or chest stiffness, the respiratory muscles must work harder to achieve the same degree of airflow. This increased work can ultimately result in respiratory muscle fatigue and respiratory failure.

© Springer International Publishing AG,
part of Springer Nature 2018
H. Poor, *Basics of Mechanical Ventilation*,
https://doi.org/10.1007/978-3-319-89981-7_8

This concept can be viewed mathematically using the equation of motion for the respiratory system, as described in Chap. 1:

$$Q = \frac{P_{air} - P_{alv}}{R}$$

P_{air} = proximal airway pressure
P_{alv} = alveolar pressure
Q = flow
R = resistance

During spontaneous breathing, the inspiratory muscles contract, causing a drop in pleural pressure, which reduces alveolar pressure. Once alveolar pressure is less than proximal airway pressure, air will flow into the patient (represented by a positive Q in the above equation). Neuromuscular weakness and increased lung or chest wall stiffness make generating low alveolar pressure more difficult. The presence of increased airway resistance necessitates even lower alveolar pressure to achieve the same inspiratory flow. If a patient is unable to sufficiently reduce alveolar pressure to achieve adequate inspiratory flow, hypoventilation and respiratory failure may develop.

Positive pressure from mechanical ventilation decreases the work of breathing by increasing proximal airway pressure. With increased proximal airway pressure, the patient needs to produce a smaller reduction in alveolar pressure to achieve the same inspiratory flow (Fig. 8.1).

Key Concept #1
Mechanical ventilation reduces work of breathing by providing the driving force for inspiration

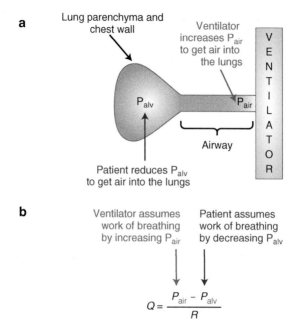

FIGURE 8.1 Diagram (**a**) and equation (**b**) of the respiratory system. The patient assumes the work of breathing during inspiration by contracting inspiratory muscles, which reduces pleural and alveolar pressure. The ventilator assumes the work of breathing during inspiration by increasing proximal airway pressure.

P_{air} proximal airway pressure; P_{alv} alveolar pressure; Q flow; R resistance

Increased airway resistance can occur not only from lower airway disorders like asthma and chronic obstructive pulmonary disease (COPD) but also from upper airway disorders such as laryngeal edema. Increased stiffness of the lungs can occur with accumulation of fluid in the lung parenchyma (cardiogenic or non-cardiogenic pulmonary edema), pulmonary infection, pulmonary hemorrhage, and pulmonary fibrosis. Increased stiffness of the chest wall can develop in kyphoscoliosis. Of note, abdominal distension, whether it be from massive ascites, obesity, or pregnancy, will increase the work of breathing because the diaphragm must expend more energy in order to descend during inspiration.

Increased Demand

Patients may develop respiratory failure in the setting of increased ventilatory demands. **Total minute ventilation**, defined as the total amount of air per unit time that enters the lungs, is equal to the product of tidal volume and respiratory rate:

$$\dot{V}_E = V_T \times RR$$

RR = respiratory rate
$\dot{V}_E$ = total minute ventilation
V_T = tidal volume

A common reason for increased demand for ventilation includes severe metabolic acidosis, in which hyperventilation is necessary for compensation of acidemia. This increased ventilatory demand is particularly problematic for patients with baseline ventilatory insufficiency like COPD or interstitial lung disease. In such cases, these patients may not be able to meet the high ventilatory requirements, ultimately developing respiratory muscle fatigue and respiratory failure.

Another cause of increased ventilatory demand is an increase in **dead-space ventilation**. Tidal volume can be partitioned into the volume of air that participates in gas exchange (**alveolar volume**) and the volume of air that does not participate in gas exchange (**dead-space volume**):

$$V_T = V_A + V_D$$

V_A = alveolar volume
V_D = dead-space volume
V_T = tidal volume

Similarly, total minute ventilation can be divided into the volume of air per unit time that participates in gas exchange (**alveolar ventilation**) and the volume of air per unit time that does not participate in gas exchange (dead-space ventilation):

$$\dot{V}_E = \dot{V}_A + \dot{V}_D$$

$\dot{V}_A$ = alveolar ventilation
$\dot{V}_D$ = dead-space ventilation
$\dot{V}_E$ = total minute ventilation

In the setting of pathology that increases dead-space ventilation, like pulmonary embolism, a patient would have to increase total minute ventilation either by increasing respiratory rate or by increasing tidal volume, in order to achieve normal alveolar ventilation.

Mechanical ventilation is also indicated for patients with severe circulatory shock, a state of decreased global oxygen delivery. The muscles of respiration require oxygen-rich blood flow in order to properly function. With quiet resting breathing, the muscles of respiration receive approximately 5% of the cardiac output; however, in states of critical illness like shock, they may receive as much as 20% of the cardiac output. With mechanical ventilation, work of breathing is taken over by the ventilator, and the respiratory muscles are unloaded. With this unloading, the muscles of respiration will require a lower percentage of the cardiac output, and blood flow will be diverted to more essential organs, such as the brain, heart, and kidneys.

Key Concept #2
Mechanical ventilation is indicated in severe circulatory shock to reduce respiratory muscle oxygen consumption

Neuromuscular Weakness

Neuromuscular weakness resulting in respiratory failure can develop secondary to acute conditions such as Guillain-Barre syndrome, chronic and relapsing conditions such as myasthenia gravis, or progressive conditions such as amyotrophic lateral sclerosis. Ventilators provide assistance by decreasing the work of breathing in these scenarios.

Alveolar Hypoventilation

As described above, alveolar ventilation is defined as the volume of air per unit time that participates in gas exchange. Arterial partial pressure of carbon dioxide ($PaCO_2$) is inversely proportional to alveolar ventilation. When alveolar ventilation is high, $PaCO_2$ is low (below 40 mm Hg). When alveolar ventilation is low, $PaCO_2$ is high (above 40 mm Hg):

$$PaCO_2 \; \alpha \; \frac{1}{\dot{V}_A}$$

Alveolar hypoventilation is defined as decreased ventilation of the gas exchanging units. This condition develops in patients who either "**won't breathe**" or "**can't breathe**."

"*Won't breathe*" refers to hypoventilation because of a decrease in respiratory drive. Common reasons for decreased respiratory drive include drug-induced sedation, central nervous system disorders, or profound systemic disorders such as circulatory shock and metabolic encephalopathy. **Apnea**, defined as the complete cessation of breathing, is the extreme form of "*won't breathe*" hypoventilation. In the setting of apnea, mechanical ventilators assume all of the work of breathing.

"*Can't breathe*" refers to hypoventilation secondary to neuromuscular weakness or conditions that increase the work of breathing. For patients with this form of hypoventilation, ventilation is difficult because of increased airway resistance, stiff lungs or chest wall, or neuromuscular weakness, leading to decreased ventilation and ultimately hypercapnia. It is important to note that severely elevated $PaCO_2$ from *"can't breathe"* can paradoxically reduce respiratory drive, adding an additional *"won't breathe"* component. This additional alveolar hypoventilation from hypercapnia is known as **CO_2 narcosis**.

> **Key Concept #3**
> Causes of alveolar hypoventilation: **won't breathe** or **can't breathe**

Alveolar hypoventilation is one of the pathophysiologic causes of hypoxemia. Additionally, elevated $PaCO_2$ results in acidemia, a condition known as **respiratory acidosis**. Mechanical ventilation can correct alveolar hypoventilation by triggering breaths for adequate ventilation in cases of *"won't breathe"* and by reducing the patient's work of breathing in cases of *"can't breathe."*

Hypoxemia

Hypoxemia is defined as a low arterial partial pressure of oxygen (PaO_2). The five pathophysiologic causes of hypoxemia include low partial pressure of inspired oxygen (P_IO_2), alveolar hypoventilation, ventilation-perfusion (V/Q) mismatch, shunt, and diffusion abnormality.

> **Key Concept #4**
> Five pathophysiologic causes of hypoxemia:
>
> - Alveolar hypoventilation
> - Low P_IO_2
> - V/Q mismatch
> - Shunt
> - Diffusion abnormality

P_IO_2 is the product of atmospheric pressure (P_{atm}) and fraction of inspired oxygen (F_IO_2):

$$P_IO_2 = F_IO_2 \times P_{atm}$$

Low P_IO_2 as the cause of hypoxemia is rare in clinical practice given that there are no clinical scenarios in which a patient is administered less than 21% F_IO_2, and hypoxemia caused by low atmospheric pressure occurs only at very high altitudes. Alveolar hypoventilation, defined as high $PaCO_2$, is described above. Ventilation-perfusion mismatch produces hypoxemia in areas of the lung where there is low ventilation relative to perfusion, such that the blood exiting that portion of the lung has low partial pressure of oxygen. Shunt is the extreme and singular point of *V/Q* mismatch, where blood passes from the venous circulation into the arterial circulation without receiving any ventilation or exchanging gas. Shunt can occur through the heart (e.g., patent foramen ovale) or lungs (e.g., pneumonia). Diffusion abnormality occurs when it takes oxygen longer than normal to diffuse from the alveolus into the blood because the alveoli are filled with a substance (e.g., edema, inflammatory cells) or because the alveolar-capillary membrane is thickened.

Mechanical ventilation is helpful because of its ability to deliver high concentrations of oxygen (high F_IO_2). Additionally, positive pressure may assist in improving gas exchange by maintaining alveolar patency.

Airway Protection

The airway is located perilously close to the esophagus, a tract through which food and oral secretions enter. The oropharynx has a number of sophisticated mechanisms that prevent food and secretions from entering the lungs. When these mechanisms are compromised, secretions can enter the lungs, leading to aspiration pneumonitis, pneumonia, and mucus plugging with resultant atelectasis. Cough, one of the lungs' most important defense mechanisms, causes the expulsion of foreign objects and secretions. Patients may be deemed as unable to "protect the airway" if there is impaired sensorium and secretion control or inability to produce an effective cough. These factors portend a risk of imminent respiratory failure. Endotracheal intubation may be necessary to assist with the clearance of secretions and to further "protect the airway" from aspiration and additional secretions.

It is important to note that many patients develop respiratory failure because of a combination of the above etiologies. For example, a patient with underlying myasthenia gravis who acutely develops septic shock and acute respiratory distress syndrome will likely have components of neuromuscular weakness, increased work of breathing, increased ventilatory demand, hypoxemia, and hypoventilation, necessitating mechancial ventilation to support gas exchange and reduce work of breathing.

Suggested Readings

1. Costanzo L. Physiology. 5th ed. Beijing: Saunders; 2014.
2. MacIntyre N, Branson R. Mechanical ventilation. 2nd ed. Philadelphia: Saunders; 2009.
3. Broaddus V, Ernst J. Murray and Nadel's textbook of respiratory medicine. 5th ed. Philadelphia: Saunders; 2010.
4. Rhoades R, Bell D. Medical physiology: principles for clinical medicine. 4th ed. Philadelphia: Lippincott Williams & Wilkins; 2013.
5. Tobin M. Principles and practice of mechanical ventilation. 3rd ed. Beijing: McGraw-Hill; 2013.
6. West J. Respiratory physiology: the essentials. 9th ed. Beijing: Lippincott Williams & Wilkins; 2012.
7. West J. Pulmonary pathophysiology: the essentials. 8th ed. Beijing: Lippincott Williams & Wilkins; 2013.

Chapter 9
Weaning from the Ventilator

While mechanical ventilation may be necessary to support ventilation and gas exchange, prolonged time on the ventilator is associated with significant complications, including lung injury, infections, and neuromuscular weakness. Therefore, in patients deemed to no longer require ventilatory support, it is important to discontinue mechanical ventilation as soon as possible. However, prematurely discontinuing mechanical ventilation may necessitate reintubation, a procedure that is associated with increased risk of adverse outcomes. The weaning process begins with an assessment of readiness to wean, followed by a diagnostic test, known as the **spontaneous breathing trial**, to determine the likelihood of successful extubation.

Assessing Readiness to Wean

Three major criteria should be fulfilled prior to initiating the weaning process:

1. Significant improvement in the initial cause of respiratory failure, either with therapy (e.g., antibiotics, diuresis, steroids) or with time (e.g., wearing off of sedation, resolution of pulmonary inflammation).

© Springer International Publishing AG, part of Springer Nature 2018
H. Poor, *Basics of Mechanical Ventilation*, https://doi.org/10.1007/978-3-319-89981-7_9

2. Adequate oxygenation with minimal F_IO_2 and PEEP. Generally accepted parameters are oxygen saturation above 90% with $F_IO_2 \leq 0.4$ and PEEP ≤ 8 cm H_2O.

3. Ability to initiate breaths spontaneously.

Other parameters that should be assessed include mental status, respiratory secretions, cough strength, respiratory demand, and cardiovascular status. A patient with depressed sensorium or poor cough strength may not adequately expel secretions to protect the airway after extubation. Retained secretions can cause mucus plugging of airways and subsequent atelectasis, leading to respiratory failure.

Patients with high ventilatory demand (e.g., significant acidemia or fever) may not be able to meet the high ventilatory requirements after extubation, resulting in post-extubation respiratory failure. This phenomenon is particularly important in patients with underlying lung disease.

As discussed in Chap. 8, mechanical ventilation is useful in states of severe circulatory shock, a state of decreased global oxygen delivery. By decreasing the patient's work of breathing, mechanical ventilation decreases the oxygen requirement of the respiratory muscles, allowing for the allotment of more cardiac output toward other essential organs such as the brain, heart, and kidneys. A patient requiring high doses of vasopressor or inotropic medications may be at high risk for decompensation after extubation as the muscles of respiration would then "steal" some of the cardiac output previously allotted to more essential organs.

Spontaneous Breathing Trial

A spontaneous breathing trial (SBT) should be conducted in patients deemed ready to wean. The SBT simulates post-extubation conditions. Its purpose is to assess whether the patient has adequate respiratory strength and stamina for the imposed respiratory load. The trial helps determine whether a patient will adequately meet ventilatory and gas exchange requirements without the assistance of mechanical ventilation. Two common ways to conduct the SBT are either using a **T-piece** or low-level pressure support ventilation (PSV) mode. SBTs usually last between thirty minutes and two hours.

Key Concept #1
Spontaneous breathing trials simulate post-extubation conditions

T-Piece Trial

A method to simulate post-extubation conditions is to simply disconnect the endotracheal tube from the ventilator. The endotracheal tube remains secured in the airway, but no positive pressure is delivered. In these cases, a T-shaped adapter ("T-piece") is connected to the endotracheal tube through which supplemental humidified oxygen is delivered. In essence, the T-piece apparatus can be viewed as a nasal cannula for the endotracheal tube (Fig. 9.1).

During this trial, the patient is monitored for signs of impending respiratory failure including tachypnea, accessory muscle use, hypoxemia, agitation or somnolence, hemodynamic changes (e.g., tachycardia, hypertension), and diapho-

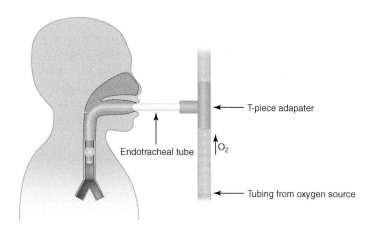

FIG. 9.1 T-piece setup. The patient is disconnected from the ventilator, but the endotracheal tube remains in the airway. A T-shaped adapter is affixed to the end of the endotracheal tube, allowing for the delivery of humidified oxygen.

resis. If significant signs of respiratory failure develop, the SBT is considered failed and is terminated by reconnecting the endotracheal to the ventilator. As the patient was not extubated, there is no need to reintubate the patient, and the risks of reintubation are avoided. The emergence of signs of respiratory failure during a T-piece trial implies that positive pressure from the ventilator is still necessary to reduce work of breathing and that without positive pressure, the patient would likely experience respiratory failure.

There are several limitations of a T-piece trial. The endotracheal tube's long, narrow lumen results in increased airway resistance compared to a normal airway. This higher resistance necessitates increased work of breathing in order to achieve the same degree of flow and ventilation, akin to breathing through a straw. Therefore, the T-piece trial may impose an unnecessarily high respiratory load and can underestimate readiness for extubation. It is important to note that airway resistance and work of breathing during a T-piece trial depend on endotracheal tube diameter. A smaller diameter endotracheal tube will require more work to achieve the same inspiratory flow compared with a larger diameter endotracheal tube.

For patients with upper airway (e.g., laryngeal) edema or obstruction, the endotracheal tube reduces resistance as it acts to stent open the upper airway. In these scenarios, work of breathing during the trial is less than after extubation, overestimating the likelihood of successful extubation. The **cuff leak test** can help predict increased airway resistance after extubation. This concept will be further explored later in this chapter.

Key Concept #2

T-piece trial:

- Patient disconnected from ventilator
- Endotracheal tube remains in airway
- Oxygen delivered via **T-piece**
- No positive pressure provided

Pressure Support Ventilation

PSV is one of the basic modes of ventilation described in Chap. 3. PSV is a patient-triggered, pressure-targeted, flow-cycled mode of ventilation. The ventilator delivers flow to quickly achieve and maintain a set proximal airway pressure, until flow depreciates to a set percentage of peak inspiratory flow. The flow waveform, tidal volume, and inspiratory time vary based on characteristics of the respiratory system and patient respiratory effort.

PSV has two characteristics that make it particularly suitable for determining the likelihood of successful extubation. First, the trigger for PSV consists only of a patient (assist) trigger and lacks the ventilator (control) trigger. Therefore, patients must be able to initiate breaths by themselves in this mode of ventilation. Second, proximal airway pressure (target) is set at a level that offsets the increased work of breathing caused by increased airway resistance of the endotracheal tube. While it is difficult to determine the exact proximal airway pressure required to offset the endotracheal tube's increased resistive load, proximal airway pressure of about 5 cm H_2O is generally used for this purpose. If a patient can generate enough inspiratory flow to achieve sufficiently high tidal volume at this low proximal airway pressure, then there is likely sufficient respiratory muscle strength for the load to breathe without mechanical ventilation.

> **Key Concept #3**
> **High tidal volume** during PSV with **low P_{air}** indicates adequate respiratory muscle strength relative to respiratory load

This concept can be further understood with the equation from Chap. 1:

$$Q = \frac{P_{air} - P_{alv}}{R}$$

P_{air} = proximal airway pressure
P_{alv} = alveolar pressure
Q = flow
R = resistance

During PSV, proximal airway pressure (target) is set by the clinician. When the patient makes an inspiratory effort, alveolar pressure decreases. To maintain proximal airway pressure at the set target, the ventilator increases flow, thereby increasing tidal volume. Imagine a patient with extremely weak respiratory muscles who cannot significantly reduce alveolar pressure with inspiratory efforts but can still trigger the ventilator. Proximal airway pressure can be set at a high level to produce inspiratory flow and tidal volume that are normal. For this patient, assume that proximal airway pressure of 20 cm H_2O leads to tidal volume of 500 mL with a respiratory rate of 10 breaths per minute. Therefore, total minute ventilation is 5 L/minute. With this high level of proximal airway pressure, the ventilator is essentially assuming all of the work of breathing. If proximal airway pressure is then reduced and the patient still cannot significantly reduce alveolar pressure because of severe weakness, the ventilator must provide less flow to maintain the lower proximal airway pressure. Therefore, tidal volume will decrease. For our patient, assume that decreasing proximal airway pressure to 5 cm H_2O leads to tidal volume of 100 mL. This decrease in tidal volume results in hypoventilation. As a compensatory response, the patient will increase his or her respiratory rate in an attempt to maintain minute ventilation. This breathing pattern of low tidal volume with a high respiratory rate is referred to as **rapid shallow breathing**. Rapid shallow breathing is a sign of respiratory weakness relative to the imposed respiratory load and suggests that extubation will likely not be tolerated. For our patient with proximal airway pressure of 5 cm H_2O who is achieving a tidal volume of 100 mL, a respiratory rate of 50 breaths per minute would be necessary to produce a minute ventilation of 5 L/minute. Even if this patient were able to reach such a high respiratory rate, he or she would not be able to maintain this rate for a sustained period and respiratory failure would recur.

Key Concept #4
Rapid shallow breathing: sign of respiratory muscle weakness relative to respiratory load

Now imagine a patient with strong respiratory muscles. If the ventilator provides normal inspiratory flow, with resultant normal tidal volume, on a setting of low proximal airway pressure (assume 5 cm H_2O), the patient is demonstrating that he or she is significantly reducing alveolar pressure with his or her own inspiratory efforts. The ability to appropriately reduce alveolar pressure with inspiratory efforts is an indication of good respiratory strength relative to respiratory load. As discussed in Chap. 8, higher inspiratory force is necessary to sufficiently reduce alveolar pressure for stiff lungs than for compliant lungs. Similarly, lower alveolar pressure must be generated to achieve adequate flow in the setting of increased airway resistance. Therefore, a patient achieving adequate tidal volume during PSV with low set proximal airway pressure will likely have the respiratory strength to sustain appropriate spontaneous ventilation after extubation.

It is crucial to appreciate that simply being on PSV does not indicate a spontaneous breathing trial. A spontaneous breathing trial with PSV requires low proximal airway pressure. PSV with high proximal airway pressure significantly decreases patient work of breathing and does not allow for proper assessment of inspiratory strength relative to respiratory load. Therefore, it is not sufficient to say that a patient "tolerates PSV." Instead, a patient on PSV with a low proximal airway pressure setting must achieve adequate tidal volume while breathing at a reasonable (i.e., not fast) respiratory rate.

Key Concept #5
P_{air} must be low if PSV is used for a SBT

Cuff Leak Test

Placement of an endotracheal tube increases airway resistance for most patients. This increase occurs because the
endotracheal tube's lumen is usually narrower than a patient's
airway. However, in patients with upper airway obstruction
(e.g., laryngeal edema), placement of an endotracheal tube
decreases airway resistance. This decrease occurs because the
endotracheal tube stents open the narrow, obstructed por-
tions of the patient's airway. Intubation itself can cause laryngeal injury and edema, leading to upper airway obstruction
after the endotracheal tube is removed, even in patients
without preexisting upper airway obstruction.

In patients with known or suspected upper airway obstruction, it is important to determine whether the airway will
remain patent after removal of the endotracheal tube; reintubation of a patient with upper airway obstruction may be
difficult and risky. The cuff leak test is a noninvasive method
that helps predict whether the airway will remain patent after
removal of the endotracheal tube.

To perform a cuff leak test, the patient is placed on
volume-controlled ventilation. When the endotracheal tube
cuff is inflated, the volume of air that returns to the ventilator
during exhalation equals the tidal volume delivered to the
patient as there is no other route for air to escape the circuit
(Fig. 9.2a). The endotracheal cuff is then deflated. If the expiratory return volume to the ventilator significantly decreases
when the cuff is deflated, a portion of the expired air is not
returning to the ventilator through the endotracheal tube but
is instead going around the endotracheal tube and out of the
patient's mouth. This "leak" implies that there is space
between the endotracheal tube and the larynx and that the
patient's airway will likely remain patent when the endotracheal tube is removed (Fig. 9.2b). When a leak is present, one
can often hear gurgling in the patient's mouth during expiration. If there is no decrease in expiratory return volume to the
ventilator (i.e., no leak), then there is no passageway for air
to exit the patient from around the endotracheal tube. In this
scenario, the endotracheal tube may be stenting open the

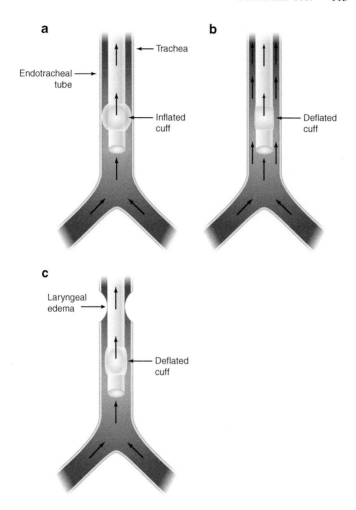

FIG. 9.2 Cuff leak test. (**a**) Because the cuff of the endotracheal tube is occluding the trachea, the entire expiratory volume goes through the endotracheal tube and back to the ventilator. Therefore, expiratory return volume is equal to tidal volume. (**b**) When the cuff is deflated, some of the expiratory volume goes around the endotracheal tube and does not return to the ventilator. Therefore, expiratory return volume is less than tidal volume. (**c**) The cuff is deflated, but because of laryngeal edema, there is no room for expiratory air to leak around the endotracheal tube. All of the expiratory volume returns to the ventilator. Therefore, expiratory return volume is equal to tidal volume.

airway, and extubation may lead to airway collapse, upper airway obstruction, and post-extubation stridor (Fig. 9.2c). While a leak can be absent in the setting of laryngeal edema or other laryngeal injuries, it can also be absent if there are secretions or if the endotracheal tube diameter is large relative to the laryngeal diameter. Therefore, the test should be considered only in patients with high risk of post-extubation stridor, such as those with a traumatic intubation or known upper airway obstruction.

Key Concept #6
Cuff leak test helps predict whether airway will remain patent after extubation

Suggested Readings

1. Boles J, Bion J, Connors A, et al. Weaning from mechanical ventilation. Eur Respir J. 2007;29:1033–56.
2. Cairo J. Pilbeam's mechanical ventilation: physiological and clinical applications. 5th ed. St. Louis: Mosby; 2012.
3. MacIntyre N, Branson R. Mechanical ventilation. 2nd ed. Philadelphia: Saunders; 2009.
4. Tobin M. Principles and practice of mechanical ventilation. 3rd ed. Beijing: McGraw-Hill; 2013.

Chapter 10
Hemodynamic Effects of Mechanical Ventilation

Critically ill patients that require mechanical ventilation often have concomitant hemodynamic instability. The direct hemodynamic effects of mechanical ventilation can further complicate their condition. Specifically, increases in intrathoracic pressure due to positive pressure ventilation can significantly impact cardiac function. It is therefore crucial to understand this interaction in order to minimize any untoward effects of mechanical ventilation.

Cardiopulmonary System

The main purpose of the cardiopulmonary system is to deliver oxygen-rich blood to the organs of the body in order to support cellular metabolism. Ventilation, the process of exchanging air within the lungs, brings oxygen to alveoli. Oxygen then diffuses into the pulmonary capillary blood. Oxygen-rich blood travels to the left side of the heart via the pulmonary veins and is ejected by the left ventricle into the systemic circulation to perfuse the body's tissues. **Stroke volume** is the amount of blood that the heart pumps out per contraction. **Cardiac output**, defined as the amount of blood

© Springer International Publishing AG,
part of Springer Nature 2018
H. Poor, *Basics of Mechanical Ventilation*,
https://doi.org/10.1007/978-3-319-89981-7_10

that the heart pumps out per unit time, is equal to the product of stroke volume and heart rate:

$$CO = SV \times HR$$

CO = cardiac output
HR = heart rate
SV = stroke volume

Note that because the right ventricle and the left ventricle are in series, right ventricular cardiac output is equal to left ventricular cardiac output in the steady state.

Oxygen in blood is present in two forms: dissolved and bound to hemoglobin. Approximately 98% of oxygen in blood is bound to hemoglobin. The remaining 2% is dissolved. **Arterial oxygen content** is the amount of oxygen bound to hemoglobin plus the amount of oxygen dissolved in arterial blood:

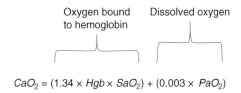

$$CaO_2 = (1.34 \times Hgb \times SaO_2) + (0.003 \times PaO_2)$$

CaO_2 = arterial oxygen content (mL of O_2 per dL of blood)
Hgb = hemoglobin (g/dL)
PaO_2 = arterial partial pressure of oxygen (mm Hg)
SaO_2 = arterial hemoglobin oxygen saturation (%)

Oxygen delivery, the amount of oxygen delivered to the body by the heart, is equal to the product of cardiac output and arterial oxygen content:

$$DO_2 = CO \times CaO_2$$

CaO_2 = arterial oxygen content
CO = cardiac output
DO_2 = oxygen delivery

Decreased oxygen delivery can be a result of decreased cardiac output (i.e., cardiogenic shock and hypovolemic shock) or a result of decreased arterial oxygen content. Decreased arterial oxygen content can occur from anemia (low hemoglobin) or hypoxemia (low PaO_2, which leads to low SaO_2). Maintaining adequate oxygen delivery is a key treatment goal in the management of critically ill patients. Therefore, it is essential to understand the effect of mechanical ventilation on cardiac output in order to prevent significant decreases in oxygen delivery.

> **Key Concept #1**
> Decreased oxygen delivery can be a result of decreased cardiac output or decreased arterial oxygen content

Intrathoracic Pressure

As discussed in Chap. 1, during spontaneous breathing, intrathoracic pressure *decreases* with inspiration. In contrast, during positive pressure ventilation, intrathoracic pressure *increases* with inspiration—the increased airway pressure is transmitted to the pleural space. The pleural space is the potential space that surrounds the lungs. The degree to which the increase in airway pressure is transmitted to the pleural space depends on lung compliance. Transmission of airway pressure is greatest when lung compliance is high (e.g., emphysema) and least when lung compliance is low (e.g., acute respiratory distress syndrome). This concept is analogous to the difference between a latex balloon and a hollow steel ball. Imagine holding a partially inflated balloon with two hands. If more air is administered into the balloon, the pressure within the balloon will increase, and the balloon will inflate. As the balloon inflates, the balloon will push your hands further apart. Because the balloon is compliant, the increase in pressure within the balloon is transmitted to your hands. Now imagine holding a hollow steel ball with two hands. If more air is administered into the steel ball, the pressure within the steel ball will increase.

However, because the walls of the steel ball are stiff and not compliant, the volume of the steel ball will not appreciably increase. Therefore, the steel ball will not push your hands further apart—in fact, your hands would probably not notice that the pressure within the steel ball had increased.

> **Key Concept #2**
> Transmission of airway pressure to the pleural space is greatest with compliant lungs and least with stiff lungs

Increases in intrathoracic pressure can result in compression of cardiac structures and intrathoracic blood vessels. This compression can lead to alterations in the loading conditions of the heart, ultimately affecting cardiac performance.

Preload

Preload is a major determinant of cardiac function. Preload is defined as the degree of ventricular stretch prior to contraction. The higher the preload, the higher the ventricular contractile force and resultant stroke volume. The relationship between preload and stroke volume is depicted by the Frank-Starling curve (Fig. 10.1). Patients existing on the steep portion of the curve are referred to as being **preload sensitive**, where small changes in preload result in large changes in stroke volume. Patients existing on the flat portion of the curve are referred to as **preload insensitive**, where changes in preload do not significantly affect stroke volume.

Mechanical ventilation decreases preload. As discussed above, positive pressure ventilation increases intrathoracic pressure. The increased intrathoracic pressure causes compression of the right heart chambers, effectively raising right

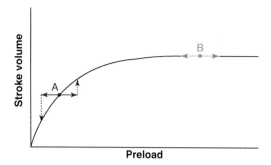

FIGURE 10.1 Frank-Starling curve. A patient at point A is preload sensitive—changes in preload lead to significant changes in stroke volume. A patient at point B is preload insensitive—changes in preload do not significantly affect stroke volume.

heart pressure. The increased right heart pressure impedes venous return to the heart, resulting in reduced end-diastolic right ventricular stretch. The decrease in right ventricular preload reduces right ventricular stroke volume, which then reduces cardiac output. As the right ventricle and left ventricle are in series, less blood is pumped to the left side of the heart, decreasing left ventricular preload. The lower left ventricular preload reduces left ventricular stroke volume and cardiac output (Fig. 10.2).

> **Key Concept #3**
> Positive pressure ventilation decreases both right and left ventricular preload

Afterload

Afterload is defined as the amount of work the heart has to do to eject blood. It is also defined as ventricular **wall stress** during systole. When the ventricular myocardium contracts,

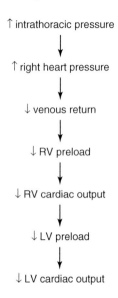

↑ intrathoracic pressure

↓

↑ right heart pressure

↓

↓ venous return

↓

↓ RV preload

↓

↓ RV cardiac output

↓

↓ LV preload

↓

↓ LV cardiac output

FIGURE 10.2 Increased intrathoracic pressure reduces preload.
RV right ventricle; *LV* left ventricle

wall stress rises, which increases ventricular pressure. The wall stress creates **transmural pressure**, which is the difference between ventricular pressure (inside the ventricle) and pericardial pressure (outside the ventricle). The sum of the forces pushing the ventricular wall outward must equal the sum of the forces pushing the ventricular wall inward. The expanding outward force is ventricular pressure. The collapsing inward forces are pericardial pressure and transmural pressure (Fig. 10.3). Note that this equilibrium is analogous to the alveolus described in Chap. 1, where alveolar pressure (outward force) is equal to the sum of pleural pressure and lung elastic recoil pressure (inward forces).

Increasing afterload shifts the Frank-Starling curve downward and to the right—stroke volume is lower for a given preload. Decreasing afterload shifts the curve upward and to the left—stroke volume is higher for a given preload (Fig. 10.4).

Increased intrathoracic pressure from positive pressure ventilation is transmitted to the pericardial space, increasing

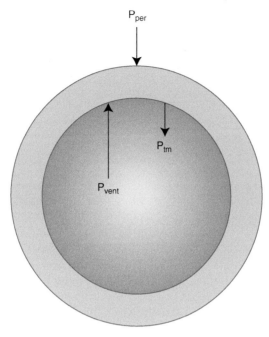

$$P_{vent} = P_{per} + P_{tm}$$

FIGURE 10.3 Diagram of a ventricular cavity. The sum of the expanding outward forces must equal the sum of the collapsing inward forces at equilibrium. Therefore, ventricular pressure equals the sum of pericardial pressure and transmural pressure.

P_{per} pericardial pressure; P_{tm} transmural pressure; P_{vent} ventricular pressure

pericardial pressure. Increased pericardial pressure reduces left ventricular afterload because the left ventricle requires a lower transmural pressure to achieve the same ventricular pressure. Imagine that pericardial pressure is 2 mm Hg. If the left ventricle needs to increase ventricular pressure to 120 mm Hg during systole, it must generate wall stress to achieve a transmural pressure of 118 mm Hg (remember $P_{tm} = P_{vent} - P_{per}$). If pericardial pressure is increased to 15 mm Hg with positive pressure ventilation, the left ventricle now needs to generate wall stress to achieve a transmural

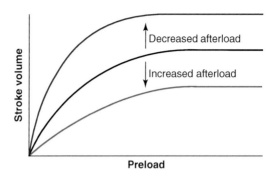

FIGURE 10.4 Frank-Starling curves demonstrating effect of changing afterload. Increasing afterload shifts the curve downward and to the right. Decreasing afterload shifts the curve upward and to the left.

pressure of only 105 mm Hg. In essence, the increased pericardial pressure around the left ventricle can be viewed as "squeezing" the left ventricle; therefore, the left ventricular myocardium has to do less work. In contrast, but by the same mechanism, the decrease in intrathoracic pressure during spontaneous breathing results in an increase in left ventricular afterload. This phenomenon is particularly evident during scenarios where intrathoracic pressure is very low during inspiration (e.g., status asthmaticus).

Key Concept #4
Positive pressure ventilation decreases left ventricular afterload

In contrast, right ventricular afterload increases with positive pressure ventilation. Within the lungs, pulmonary capillaries course adjacent to the alveoli. Gas exchange occurs at this interface between alveoli and pulmonary capillaries. Elevated alveolar pressure from positive pressure ventilation can lead to compression of pulmonary capillaries, which increases the resistance of the pulmonary vasculature. Increased pulmonary vascular resistance increases the

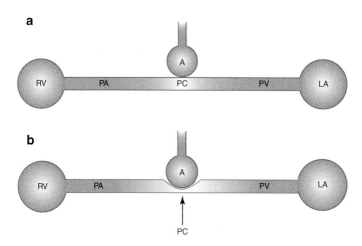

FIGURE 10.5 Schematic of the pulmonary vasculature. (**a**) The pulmonary capillaries course by alveoli. (**b**) With alveolar distension from positive pressure ventilation, the pulmonary capillaries can become compressed, increasing pulmonary vascular resistance and right ventricular afterload.

A alveolus; *LA* left atrium; *PA* pulmonary artery; *PC* pulmonary capillary; *PV* pulmonary vein; *RV* right ventricle

amount of work the right ventricle must do to eject blood; therefore, right ventricular afterload is increased (Fig. 10.5).

> **Key Concept #5**
> Positive pressure ventilation increases right ventricular afterload

Specific Hemodynamic Conditions

As evident from the prior sections in this chapter, the interplay between positive pressure ventilation and hemodynamics are multifaceted and complex. Ultimately, the effect of mechanical ventilation on cardiac function will vary, depending on the underlying hemodynamic condition.

Hypovolemia

Hypovolemia is a state of low circulating blood volume. This low blood volume results in low preload, placing patients on the preload-sensitive portion of the Frank-Starling curve, where changes in preload lead to significant changes in stroke volume (Point A in Fig. 10.1). As further decreases in preload can ensue with positive pressure ventilation, mechanical ventilation can significantly reduce stroke volume in hypovolemic patients. Many patients with hypovolemia (e.g., hemorrhage) are already in a precarious hemodynamic state — a reduction in cardiac output from mechanical ventilation may precipitate or worsen shock. Prompt and adequate fluid administration to counteract the preload reduction from positive pressure ventilation is often necessary.

Left Ventricular Failure

Patients with left ventricular failure (both systolic and diastolic dysfunction) often have high left-sided filling pressures and are in a state of volume overload, particularly in the setting of acute illness. High left-sided filling pressures lead to increased pulmonary capillary pressures, which can result in cardiogenic (hydrostatic) pulmonary edema. Additionally, volume overload results in high preload, placing these patients on the preload-insensitive portion of the Frank-Starling curve, where changes in preload do not significantly affect stroke volume (Point B in Fig. 10.1). Preload reduction is a fundamental therapeutic goal in the management of decompensated left ventricular failure. It decreases left-sided filling pressures, which decreases pulmonary capillary pressure and improves pulmonary edema. Positive pressure ventilation is helpful in patients with high left-sided filling pressures because it reduces preload without significantly affecting cardiac output, as they are often on the preload-insensitive portion of the Frank-Starling curve.

Patients with left ventricular systolic failure are particularly sensitive to changes in left ventricular afterload—increases in afterload will cause significant decreases in stroke volume and cardiac output. Positive pressure ventilation can improve hemodynamics for these patients as it decreases left ventricular afterload. As detailed above, the increased pericardial pressure helps to "squeeze" the left ventricle and reduces myocardial work.

Cardiogenic pulmonary edema occurs when high pulmonary capillary hydrostatic pressure results in transudation of fluid into the interstitium and alveoli. Pulmonary capillary pressure is often high in the setting of left ventricular failure. In addition to its beneficial effects on left ventricular preload and afterload, positive pressure ventilation increases alveolar pressure, which reduces the pressure gradient between the alveolus and the pulmonary capillary. As a result of the reduced pressure gradient, there is less transudation of fluid into the alveolus (Fig. 10.6).

For intubated patients with left ventricular failure, the beneficial effects of positive pressure ventilation on preload, after-

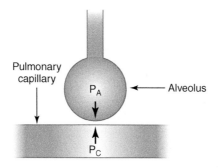

FIGURE 10.6 Relationship between pulmonary capillary pressure and alveolar pressure in the development of cardiogenic (hydrostatic) pulmonary edema. When alveolar pressure is increased due to positive pressure ventilation, the pressure gradient between the pulmonary capillary and the alveolus is reduced, decreasing fluid transudation into the alveolus.

P_A alveolar pressure; P_C pulmonary capillary pressure

load, and alveolar-capillary fluid dynamics should be taken into account when considering discontinuation of mechanical ventilation. These beneficial effects are still present during spontaneous breathing trials that use pressure support ventilation because the ventilator provides positive pressure. Extubation and discontinuation of positive pressure ventilation will result in an acute rise in left ventricular preload and afterload, as well as an increase in the capillary-alveolar pressure gradient. These changes can precipitate or exacerbate left ventricular failure and pulmonary edema. Therefore, spontaneous breathing trials using pressure support ventilation may not adequately simulate the post-extubation respiratory workload. Patients requiring ventilatory support for left ventricular dysfunction should have optimal cardiac loading conditions prior to extubation, ensuring euvolemia with diuresis and good control of systemic blood pressure. A T-piece trial (Chap. 9) does not use positive pressure and may therefore better simulate post-extubation cardiac loading conditions.

Pulmonary Hypertension and Right Ventricular Failure

Patients with pulmonary hypertension and right ventricular failure have increased right ventricular afterload. Additional increases in right ventricular afterload with positive pressure ventilation can significantly exacerbate this condition. Preload is also reduced with positive pressure ventilation, which can further decrease cardiac output (Fig. 10.7). While it is important to limit airway pressures and lung volumes during mechanical ventilation in these patients, it is equally important to avoid the deleterious consequences from atelectasis and hypoxia. Hypoxia is a strong stimulus for pulmonary vasoconstriction, which increases right ventricular afterload. Ideally, intubation and mechanical ventilation would be avoided in patients with severe pulmonary hypertension and right ventricular failure, but if mechanical ventilation is absolutely necessary, care must be taken to limit and counteract the adverse hemodynamic consequences.

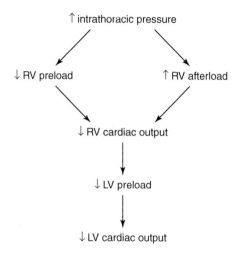

FIGURE 10.7 Increased intrathoracic pressure affects right ventricular loading conditions, leading to decreased cardiac output. *RV* right ventricle; *LV* left ventricle

Suggested Readings

1. Mann D, Zipes D. Braunwald's heart disease: a textbook of cardiovascular medicine. 10th ed. Philadelphia: Saunders; 2009.
2. Cairo J. Pilbeam's mechanical ventilation: physiological and clinical applications. 5th ed. St. Louis: Mosby; 2012.
3. Costanzo L. Physiology. 5th ed. Beijing: Saunders; 2014.
4. MacIntyre N, Branson R. Mechanical ventilation. 2nd ed. Philadelphia: Saunders; 2009.
5. Marino P. Marino's the ICU book. 3rd ed. Philadelphia: Lippincott Williams & Wilkins; 2007.
6. Poor H, Ventetuolo C. Pulmonary hypertension in the intensive care unit. Prog Cardiovasc Dis. 2012;55(2):187–98.
7. Rhoades R, Bell D. Medical physiology: principles for clinical medicine. 4th ed. Philadelphia: Lippincott Williams & Wilkins; 2013.
8. Tobin M. Principles and practice of mechanical ventilation. 3rd ed. Beijing: McGraw-Hill; 2013.

Index

© Springer International Publishing AG,
part of Springer Nature 2018
H. Poor, *Basics of Mechanical Ventilation*,
https://doi.org/10.1007/978-3-319-89981-7

132   Index